# Embracing Recovery from Chemical Dependency

## *A Personal Recovery Plan*

M. Deborah Corley, Ph.D.

Jennifer Schneider, M.D., Ph.D.

Richard Irons, M.D.

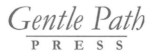

*Gentle Path*
PRESS

GENTLE PATH PRESS
P.O. Box 12863
Scottsdale, AZ 85267-2863
www.gentlepath.com
(800) 955-9853

**Embracing Recovery from Chemical Dependency**
*A Personal Recovery Plan*

Library of Congress Cataloging-in-Publication Data

Corley, M. Deborah.
  Embracing Recovery from Chemical Dependency: a
personal recovery plan / M. Deborah Corley, Jennifer P. Schneider,
Richard M. Irons.
      p. cm.
ISBN 1-929866-05-4
1. Twelve-step programs. 2. Compulsive behavior. 3. Alcoholics--Rehabilitation.
4. Narcotic addicts--Rehabilitation. I.
Schneider, Jennifer P. II. Irons, Richard, M.D. III. Title.
BF632.C63 2003
616.86'0651--dc21                                      2003000434

Publisher
Shari Jo Hehr

Editor
Sally M. Scott

Interior Design
Kim Eoff

Cover Design
Tammie Oldham

Author's note: The stories in this book are true; however, each has been edited for clarity. Names, locations, and other identifying information have been changed to protect confidentiality.

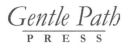

*Although Richard Irons is greatly missed by family, friends, colleagues, and the recovery community, we dedicate this book to the ones who miss him most—his wife Kirsten, and his children, Hillary, Trevor, Lee Thomas, and Ethan.*

–Deb, Jennifer, Pat, and Shari Jo

# Gentle Path Press Books

## Available

### Open Hearts
Patrick Carnes, Ph.D., Debra, Laaser, and Mark Laaser, Ph.D.

### Facing the Shadow
Patrick Carnes, Ph.D.

### Cybersex Unhooked
David Delmonico, Ph.D., Elizabeth Griffin, M.A., and Joseph Moriarity

### Disclosing Secrets
Jennifer Schneider, M.D., Ph.D., and M. Deborah Corley, Ph.D.

### Embracing Recovery from Chemical Dependency
M. Deborah Corley, Ph.D., Jennifer Schneider, M.D., Ph.D., and Richard Irons, M.D.
*Summer, 2003*

---

## Upcoming Publications

### Sex, Lies, and Forgiveness, 2nd Ed.
*Jennifer P. Schneider, M.D.*

### Back from Betrayal, 2nd Ed.
*Jennifer P. Schneider, M.D.*

www.GentlePath.com   (800) 955-9853

# Gentle Path Video and Audio Resources

## Contrary to Love: Helping the Sexual Addict

Tape 1: Our Addictive Society

Tape 2: Cultural Denial of Addiction

Tape 3: Am I an Addict?

Tape 4: Interview with Three Addicts

Tape 5: The Addictive Family

Tape 6: Interview with Melody Beattie

Tape 7: Child Abuse

Tape 8: The Twelve-Step Recovery Process

Tape 9: Healthy Sexuality and Spirituality

Tape 10: Finding a Balance in Recovery

Tape 11: Coping in a World of Shame

Tape 12: The Ten Risks of Recovery

Video (1 hour each). You may order individual tapes or the entire set.

Audio (12 tape set only – 1 hour each)

## Trauma Bonds: When We Bond to Those Who Hurt Us

Video (1 hour)

Audio (4 tape set – 90 minutes each)

## Addiction Interaction Disorder: Understanding Multiple Addictions

Video (1 hour)

Audio (1 hour)

## Toward a New Freedom: Discovering Healthy Sexuality

Audio (2 hours)

## Sexual Abuse in the Church

Audio (1 hour)

## Sexual Dependency, Compulsion, and Obsession

Audio (4 tape set – 90 minutes each)

**www.GentlePath.com   (800) 955-9853**

# Table of Contents

# Preface

This book began as the inspiration and writing of our friend and colleague, Dr. Richard Irons. Richard began his professional career as a physician in the field of internal medicine. Later, like so many other physicians, Richard became active in addiction medicine after years of recovering from his own chemical dependency. At first he worked with physicians recovering from drug addiction, and later he became a leader in diagnosing and treating professionals who were suffering from addictive sexual disorders and from multiple addictions.

In March 2002, while Richard was working on this book, he died unexpectedly, apparently from an abnormal heart rhythm.

We undertook to finish this project. In his original preface, Richard wrote:

> In the idealistic and stormy days of my adolescence, I had many dreams and aspirations, but I never once thought that I would become addicted to a drug.
>
> I discovered that the magical and mystical power I attached to this substance would challenge the bonds I treasured to my family, my profession, and God. I woke up to find that I was unable to help myself and unwilling to believe I could trust anyone with my secrets.
>
> I knew I had to change how I lived in the world. This was the only way I would experience what it was like to once again be truly free, content, and able to choose each day to honor and marvel at the wonder of life as it lives itself in everyone and everything around me and within me.

With this book, Richard hoped to help other addicts experience the joy and wonder of life he found as a recovering person. We wish the same for you.

This book is not just something for you to read passively. It is a workbook, meaning that you will get the most out of it if you actively participate by giving thoughtful attention to the questions we pose to you and then by writing down your answers. We encourage you to keep a companion journal to record your emotional responses while working on a particular chapter or exercise. You may also want to use your journal to write down additional thoughts as you go through the chapters of this book.

The chapters are arranged in a logical order, first determining how using alcohol or other drugs has solved or created problems in your life and then breaking through the denial of your addiction (Chapter One), understanding the nature of the disease of addiction (Chapter Two), recognizing how addiction affected you personally, (Chapter Three), becoming ready to begin the process of recovery (Chapter Four), recognizing the physical costs of your addiction (Chapter Five) and its damage to your relationships, career, and soul, and how to disclose your behaviors (Chapter Six), developing victim empathy and becoming accountable (Chapter Seven), defining your own sobriety and learning how to stay motivated while you practice basic recovery skills (Chapter Eight), creating a community to support your recovery (Chapter Nine), preparing for and preventing relapse (Chapter Ten), and maintaining long-term recovery (Chapter Eleven). We have included an appendix containing the answers to frequently asked questions about addiction and recovery and another that provides recovery resources.

This is not a book to simply read through and put down forever. When you finish the last exercise, you will have a tailor-made plan specific to your own recovery. We recommend that you keep the book available, and reread relevant chapters as specific issues come up again. This book can continue helping you for a long time. Happy reading and writing! And happy recovery!

—Deborah Corley and Jennifer Schneider

# CHAPTER ONE: Denial and Other Forms of Brain Trickery

**denial** n. *a refusal to believe or accept*

# Why People Use Drugs—The Brain's Mind-Body Connection

Many people ask, "What makes people use drugs?" The truth is, people usually use drugs because they want to change how they feel. When we ask those in treatment this question, we get a resounding, "IT FEELS GOOD!" People also use drugs to be more creative, to fit in, to build self-esteem, to get a boost of courage or energy, to calm down, to demonstrate love, as a form of hatred, for money, to get back at their parents or someone in authority, to stop the noise in their head, to prove they can, because the drugs are available, and to get rid of shame and guilt.

Depending on how you want to feel, different drugs can influence brain chemistry in various ways. Using such drugs changes the messages the brain receives and presto, magic—you feel different and your behavior changes. Actually, drugs change the way we perceive and then respond to whatever is causing us emotional or in some cases physical distress. Drugs change brain chemistry. Sometimes the changes are such that people seem to like being around you more, or you seem to be more creative or clever—at least at the start. That is the unfortunate thing about drugs: In the beginning they seem to solve a problem, but over time the drug that was initially so wonderful now drives people away. Moreover, with repeated use it usually takes a larger quantity or more frequent use of the drug for the desired result to happen. You become less motivated and depressed or you get more irritated and angry or out of control in ways that cause you problems. Then people nag, or threaten to leave or throw you out, or they give you driving tickets or arrest you. All just because you were trying to find a solution to some problem life has thrown your way.

## Addicts Have a Low Emotional IQ

Addicts use drugs because they can't tolerate emotional distress. The distress may be due to psychological problems, poor coping skills, or physical pain. (Physical pain is usually associated with emotional distress, and in such cases the drug is used to relieve both the physical and the psychological pain.) A person who can't tolerate emotional distress has what is called *poor emotional competence* or *low emotional IQ*. Because such people can't stand how they feel, they drink something, snort something, shoot something, swallow something, or smoke something in order to feel different. Let's face it, if you want to change how you feel, there are plenty of drugs that do that. Drugs do make emotional pain go away—for a while. Drugs do make it possible to ignore reality—for a while. Drugs do alter mood—for a while.

Mood alteration is nothing new. We humans are driven to want to alter our moods. Babies suck their thumbs to alter their mood—to self-soothe. We might identify this thumb sucking as a healthy form of self-soothing for a baby. However, it becomes problematic if the baby never gives it up or never learns other ways to self-soothe; it is not socially appropriate for adults to sit around sucking their thumbs. Babies also rock themselves as a form of self-soothing, but an adult who exhibits such behavior as his or her only coping strategy is usually one who is mentally ill.

Babies (and adults) also alter their mood with other people. A baby who lives in a healthy, functional family might feel distress and might cry loudly for her mother. When Mom appears and soothes her with soft talking, cuddling, or a soothing touch, the baby's brain chemistry is actually changed. Adults can do this by talking or just being with some friends, by praying or meditating, and by listening to music. The resulting alterations in brain chemistry change how we perceive and then respond to the environment around us.

# Genetics, Environment, and the Luck of the Draw

Brain chemistry can also be altered by detrimental behaviors. In children and adults who have been exposed to various forms of abuse in early formative years, brain-mapping research has found differences in brain formation and electrical activity (brain chemistry in motion). When a baby who cries, hoping to get a supportive adult to nurture and soothe him, instead gets an angry, punishing adult or is totally ignored for long periods, his brain chemistry is changed as well, but not in good ways. As he gets older, such a child is likely to respond to the environment around him in unhealthy ways.

The human body manufactures certain chemicals to help transmit, block, speed up, or slow down electrical messages sent to and from the brain in response to stimuli. These chemicals are called *neurochemicals* or *neurotransmitters*. Some examples are dopamine, epinephrine, norepinephrine, serotonin, and glutamate. Genetics play a role in how your brain is formatted—and in the way the brain uses these chemicals. Certain gene combinations predispose people to addiction as well as to various conditions related to neurochemical imbalances such as depression, bipolar disease, and anxiety disorders. Genetic factors can at least in part explain why addiction and some psychiatric disorders run in families. Often, however, it is not clear to researchers what comes first, the neurochemical imbalance or the environment that worsens problems with neurochemical imbalances.

In addition to genetics, your chance of being an addict is strongly influenced by the family you grew up in. Family (or those folks who take care—or don't take care—depending on your luck of the draw) plays a huge role in how you learn to adapt to the environment around you and how your emotional competency is developed. This emotional competency is related to how you respond to neurochemical imbalances as well. The more emotionally competent you become, the more you are able to motivate yourself to control your impulses, delay gratification, and self-soothe in healthy ways. Family is the first teacher of the skills associated with emotional competence.

Your family experiences greatly influence what you grow up believing about yourself as well. As you became a teenager and then an adult, you came to believe things about yourself based on what you were exposed to during your childhood years. These core beliefs constantly speak to the child (and later the adult) about how to think about oneself in a situation. For the addict, these core beliefs include "I am not a worthwhile person," "no one would love me if they really knew me," "I can't rely on anyone else," and "my [addictive] drug or behavior is my most important need." Such unhealthy beliefs are what fuel the addictive system.

Poor emotional competence results in an inability to cope with the feelings associated with that set of core beliefs. As we stated earlier, this inability to tolerate emotional distress is what drives an addict to use drugs.

Most of our methods of coping also have their beginnings in our childhood. Depending on your genetic makeup and your experiences, your drug of choice for coping is usually related to how you learned to cope as a kid. For example, if you used fantasy to escape, you are more likely to look for drugs that allow you to escape: Hallucinogens (mushrooms, LSD, PCP), natural psychedelics like peyote, or cannabis (marijuana) might be the drugs that work best to help you cope. Perhaps you were someone who, as a child, coped with feelings of unworthiness by endlessly watching TV or bingeing on food. You might choose a depressant such as heroin or other narcotics to shut out the negative feelings by reducing stimulation from those internal or external demons. You might also use alcohol or sedatives of some sort. The basic motivation is satiation to avoid stimulation and confrontation.

Other folks choose just the opposite route. They want high arousal to make themselves feel better. As kids, these high-risk takers were the first to steal a toy out of spite or ride their bikes without training wheels—*down the street and across the highway*! They are the first to try bungee jumping or sky-diving or rock climbing. As teens or in adulthood, they seek stimulant drugs such as amphetamines or cocaine for the arousal state. They usually smoke or chew tobacco and drink large quantities of coffee or colas with caffeine. They often use their drug of choice just before or while engaging in high-risk behavior such as gambling, shoplifting, or sexually cheating on their partner. When the environment seems overwhelming or challenging in some way, they feel an urge to be energetic and powerful. These folks often have a history of impulsiveness that results in life-threatening events.

# Using This Workbook as a Tool for Clarity and Change

One way that healthy people gain clarity about a situation is to write about it. Journaling has long been known to be a wonderful way to self-soothe. Instead of obsessing about your thoughts and feelings or "stuffing" them some place in your head, you are able to sort them out and leave them on the paper. In contrast, "stuffing" keeps you confused, angry, resentful, or afraid. We invite you to pick up your pen and actually write in this workbook or a journal if you need more space. You may need to keep the information private until you and a therapist can determine what is important to share for your recovery (and for the well-being and safety of others).

# Description of an Addict

Most people who read this book have been told by someone that they are an addict or they are worried they might have a problem. Perhaps that is true for you. If you are like us, you have your own description of an addict. It is one that you are using to measure your own behavior against to determine if you are addict. You might find it helpful to get clear about that description now.

## Exercise 1:   My Description of an Addict

Take a few moments to complete the following exercise to refer back to later in the book. You may find it helpful to keep the information in your own personal journal until you are ready to share it with someone else. Or you may want to just jot down the answers in the space provided below.

_____

_____

_____

_____

_____

_____

Try to form a mental picture of a real or imaginary person you consider to be an alcoholic or drug addict, a person who is the same age, race, and gender as you.

Write down this description in your journal or below. If it helps, draw a picture (You do not have to be an artist!), or use symbols or objects that you associate with an alcoholic or someone addicted to another drug. Include some words that fall into the following categories:

- Beliefs about themselves, about other people, about the world in general

- Attitudes about their use of the drug

- Patterns of using the drug

- When and where they use the drug

- Appearance when under the influence

- Behaviors when under the influence compared to when they aren't using

- Problems caused by the person's drug use

- Things put aside or given up in order to continue using drugs

Write the description here:

_____

_____

_____

Draw a picture here:

Stop for a minute and reflect upon your efforts. How is the description of an addict related to how you view yourself?

_____

_____

_____

_____

How is the description similar to what others have told you about yourself?

_____

_____

_____

_____

# No One Wants to Be an Addict

No one wants to be an addict. It is not one of those things you hold your hand up and volunteer for. It just sneaks up on you: One day, someone complains about how much you drink, or suggests that you are using too much of some other drug and that it is ruining your life. You feel you have to construct an elaborate story about how much you can handle or a defense that the amount you use isn't that much—that you can control it. You know the famous line, "I can stop anytime I want to." These accusers don't know what they are talking about! Just look, you can go to work and get your job done, no problem. In fact, you pride yourself on how clever you are in getting the money you use to buy drugs or how much you can get done when you are using.

Besides, you have good reasons to use. If your husband would just help a little more with the kids and stop complaining about what a mess the house is after he works so hard at his important job, maybe you wouldn't need to take that extra Lortab pill to get through the day. If you didn't have to work such long hours or meet that short deadline, you wouldn't need the extra punch that the amphetamines so seductively provide. If your wife wasn't so frigid and would just put out a little more often, you won't be enticed by that topless bar and the half-dozen drinks you have to reduce your guilt and inhibition with the lap dancer while you fantasize that she will solve your problems. If you could just find the right man who would want you for something besides just sex, you might not need the heroin to take away the pain of feeling so worthless and hopeless about your life.

Then one day suddenly you find that you used more than you intended to use, or you spent money on your drug when you needed to use that money for rent or groceries or your daughter's braces. Or perhaps you realize you've spent hours thinking about how you are going to get that drug, or what it will feel like, or you actually spend more hours than you intended just getting the drug. Not to mention the time it takes now to recover from several hours or days of using. What finally grabs your attention is when you find you are on the other side of a binge and you know that your wife has already said she will move out if you shoot up again. Or your Dad said he would not bail you out of jail again and now you have another DWI. Or you have lost your job because you failed the random drug screen, but you can't stop yourself from using and you don't know how to go home and face your family.

## Exercise 2:  My Personal Relationship with Drugs

If you are like most folks with a drug problem, you have formed a relationship with mood-altering drugs. One important task is to look at how they help(ed) you.

Start with your history. The exercise that follows will assist you in remembering the history of how you came to use and then to be dependent upon your drug of choice (and the drugs that you substitute if your favorite drug is unavailable).

The questions below will help you remember the story of how you were introduced and began to use drugs. The process is designed to help you think about the stages of forming your relationship with drugs—all of them along the way. (That includes nicotine, so indicate how cigarette or tobacco use is a part of this. Research has shown that nicotine helps the brain stay stuck in the "I want to use my drug!" screaming mode.)

Read through the questions first, then take some time to think about the answers. If you like, you can answer the questions one by one in your journal; then, using that information, write the story below about your personal relationship with your drugs. This is a story that you will be able to tell your therapist and that will be very helpful for both of you in creating a relapse-prevention plan.

Feel free to write more information that comes to mind. (Caution: If you find that you are getting into what we term "euphoric recall"—remembering all the positive effects to such an extent that you want to go use—then it would be wise for you to seek the help of a therapist and to get to a twelve step meeting if you haven't yet done this. See the Resource Appendix at the end of the book for information about how to find a meeting, locate a therapist, get a sponsor, and so on. Another technique for reducing craving or urges is located in Chapter Eleven. Use every tool you can to help yourself—you deserve to get your life back!)

# Here Are the Questions:

1.  What mood-altering drug do you consider your substance of choice?

    _____

2.  What was the first mood-altering drug you began using?

    _____

3.  Can you recall the first time you saw someone use or be intoxicated and under the influence of this drug or how you discovered it? Any thoughts about the person who used it then and now? Who was it? How old were you?

    _____

    _____

    _____

    _____

4.  Are there any other people whose use of this substance made a distinct impression on you?

    _____

    _____

5. What movies or television programs do you recall in which the use of this drug was glamorized or romanticized? Did they make the use of it seem attractive? Did you see these programs before or after you first used the substance?

_____

_____

_____

6. Did one or perhaps several people you knew describe how this drug made them feel, or tell you stories about what they did while they were using? Who, if anyone, wanted you to try this drug for the first time, or with whom you were involved during the early stage of your use?

_____

_____

_____

7. What books, Internet sites, or other information influenced your decision to try this substance?

_____

_____

_____

8. What special or personal names have you used to refer to this substance?

_____

_____

_____

9. When and where did you first use this substance? Did you combine it with any other drugs the first time you used?

_____

_____

_____

10. Describe the day, who were you with, and what were you doing.

_____

_____

_____

11. How did the experience make you feel? Any side effects during or after use?

_____

_____

_____

12. How did it help you? What did it solve or provide for you during the first use?

_____

_____

_____

13. Do you believe you used this drug to excess on this first encounter?

_____

_____

_____

14. Can you remember the details of any other early drug use that seem important to note?

_____

_____

_____

15. What occasions during your early use (the first ten times or first year of using) had special significance? Were there any important life experiences or events while "under the influence?"

_____

_____

_____

16. How did your drug use affect the major areas of your life, such as work, family, religious practice, hobbies, favorite activities, ability to make friends, time with old friends, or other areas of interest?

_____

_____

_____

17. What changes in your appearance, dress, interests, friends, and activities do you recall?

_____

_____

_____

18. When did you first begin to shift your focus in life more toward your relationship with this drug than your relationship with your family, work, or other important things in your life? At what point did you know that the drugs had "moved in"—when you thought they would always be available and would always be willing to help you change the way you feel?

_____

_____

_____

19. How has your drug use changed? When did the drugs begin to falter in solving problems for you and begin to be the problem? In what

ways did your preoccupation with getting more or changing your use increase in hopes of capturing that first incredible high again?

_____

_____

_____

20. When, where, and how much do you use now?

_____

_____

_____

21. On which occasions have you used too much at any time or for too long? Describe how you experienced loss of control.

_____

_____

_____

22. What are the longest periods of time that you have not used any mood-altering drugs? What motivated you to stop using for that period of time?

_____

_____

_____

23. Describe any frightening or unpleasant feelings associated with drug use.

_____

_____

_____

24. Does this drug have the same effect on you now as it did one year ago? Five years ago?

_____

_____

25. What has changed?

_____

_____

_____

Now write your story about your relationship with drugs. Be as honest with yourself as you can.

_____

_____

_____

_____

_____

_____

_____

_____

_____

_____

_____

_____

_____

_____

_____

_____

_____

_____

_____

_____

# Excuses, Secrets, Problems, and Consequences

Making excuses for using drugs when you can't cope with a situation is a real sign of denial. Another is pretending there are no problems in your life as a result of using. The extent to which you lie and keep secrets reflects how life has become unmanageable because the more you lie and keep secrets, the more you have to lie to protect the secret. It becomes a vicious cycle. The exercises below will help you gain awareness that can be one of the most important steps of beginning to change your life. The more honest you can be here, the more you increase your chances for success.

In the paragraphs above we mentioned some excuses people use to use. Let's take a look at how you have convinced yourself that it is okay for you to use, that you deserve it, that it isn't so bad.

## Exercise 3:   Twenty Excuses I Use to Use

In the spaces below, write twenty of your favorite ways you tell yourself it is okay or you deserve to use drugs. These excuses are how you lie to yourself.

1. _____
2. _____
3. _____
4. _____
5. _____
6. _____
7. _____
8. _____
9. _____
10. _____
11. _____
12. _____
13. _____
14. _____

15. _____

16. _____

17. _____

18. _____

19. _____

20. _____

The truth is, if you are making excuses like those you've listed, you probably cannot control your drug use the way you thought you could. If you could, it wouldn't be hard to quit. The thought of quitting wouldn't be so scary. People wouldn't be complaining. You wouldn't have the problems you now face.

If you really want to get honest with yourself, help yourself recognize the problems that have grown out of your drug use. Completing the next exercise will help you begin to see how your drug use has started to control your life.

## Exercise 4:   Problems List

The exercises you have completed up to now have presented a snapshot of your life up to the present. If you are to this point, someone or your own conscience has been pointing out that your drug use has caused you problems. It is important to acknowledge those and get clear about what secrets and lies are attached to the problems. This will help you stay focused on what is important to you as you begin this process of change. Making a list of your current problems will help your therapist and probably save you some therapy dollars because you can bring this information already complete to a therapy session. If you aren't seeing a therapist, the list will be a great way for you to see clear evidence of why the relationship with your drug of choice is troublesome. It will give others who are crucial in your recovery a way to know you are serious about making changes in your life.

Remember that you are making this list for yourself. It helps you to put in perspective where you are and where you want to be. At first, it may feel uncomfortable or discouraging to make this list. Please remember that everyone has problems, whether they are fighting an addiction or not.

List all of your problems here. Include both those that are associated with substance use and those that are not.

**Problem One:** _____

_____

_____

_____

**Problem Two:** _____

_____

_____

**Problem Three:** _____

_____

_____

_____

**Problem Four:** _____

_____

_____

_____

**Problem Five:** _____

_____

_____

_____

Problem Six:

_____

_____

_____

_____

Problem Seven:

_____

_____

_____

_____

Problem Eight:

_____

_____

_____

_____

Problem Nine:

_____

_____

_____

_____

Problem Ten:

_____

_____

_____

_____

Problem Eleven: _____

_____

_____

_____

Problem Twelve: _____

_____

_____

_____

# Secrets and Lies

Addicts are known to lie, cheat, and steal. It is a part of your double life. One part tries to be what other people want you to be and what your values and principles say you should be. The other part lurks about in shame and fear of discovery. This part has many secrets and lies.

These secrets become problems in and of themselves, engendering additional difficulties for you. After a time, it is difficult to remember who you told what. Lying then becomes part of the preoccupation. "What did I tell her about where I was?" "How do I cover up spending all this money?" You can easily trip yourself up. You may have told some lies so many times that you half believe they are the truth. After a while, you don't even know what is a lie and you begin to lie about things that aren't even related to your drug use.

Sooner or later you will hear the statement that "our secrets keep us sick." Whether or not you like this little pearl of wisdom, it is true. As the _Big Book of Alcoholics Anonymous_ says, "half measures" will not be sufficient. This is especially important to remember as you make your list of secrets and the lies you've told to keep them. Do a thorough housecleaning. The most important secrets to put down on paper are the ones buried deepest in your heart.

# Exercise 5:   My Secrets

List your secrets, from whom you keep the truth, the lie you told to hide the secret (including intimidating the other person or blaming them as a way to distract them from the issues), and the fears you wish to avoid facing by maintaining the secrets.

Examples:

## Secret

Drink secretly

## Lie I told to whom

To wife—"I don't feel well. You go to the dinner without me."

## Fear

Wife will think I am alcoholic and leave me

## Secret

I've spent all our savings on cocaine.

## Lie I told to whom

To wife—"We got another tax bill, so I had to take it out of our savings. I don't know why you are so upset. I didn't really lie. I didn't want you to worry. I was just trying to protect you."

## Fear

We won't have the money to really pay the taxes. The penalties will be so high we will never get out from under the burden and our son won't be able to go to college. Wife will think I am a failure.

## Secret

Was arrested for third DWI and am to go to court. The man I am having affair with bailed me out of jail.

## Lie I told to whom

To husband—"I was just trying to comfort Julie. She had had more to drink than me and she bailed me out. She will go to court with me; you don't need to bother."

## Fear

Husband will leave me if he finds out about the affair.

### Secret

Stole my sister's painkiller from her medicine cabinet.

### Lie I told to whom

Never told wife of past drug habit. Told her my dentist gave them to me for my toothache. Never said anything to sister.

### Fear

Wife will think I am weak if I admit I am hooked. My sister will know I have relapsed and force me into treatment.

### Secret

Stole the money from the church pancake breakfast and blamed it on the teens who worked at the breakfast.

### Lie I told to whom

To everyone—"I just discovered the money missing after those boys who were cleaning were in here."

### Fear

Everyone will think I am a loser if I admit I am a thief.

As you develop your list of secrets, note which ones are associated with your self-image, and also which ones are associated in some way with getting or using your substance.

Do you notice any patterns involving your preoccupation with your drug? How does it affect your choices? How much energy do you put into covering up, isolating, or worrying about someone finding out about your secret life?

### First Secret:

_____

_____

### Lie I told and to whom

_____

_____

_____

**Fear**

_____

_____

_____

**Second Secret**

_____

_____

**Lie I told and to whom**

_____

_____

_____

**Fear**

_____

_____

_____

**Third Secret**

_____

_____

**Lie I told and to whom**

_____

_____

_____

**Fear**

_____

_____

_____

## Fourth Secret

_____

_____

_____

## Lie I told and to whom

_____

_____

_____

## Fear

_____

_____

_____

## Fifth Secret

_____

_____

## Lie I told and to whom

_____

_____

_____

## Fear

_____

_____

_____

## Sixth Secret

_____

_____

_____

**Lie I told and to whom**

_____

_____

_____

**Fear**

_____

_____

_____

**Seventh Secret**

_____

_____

**Lie I told and to whom**

_____

_____

_____

**Fear**

_____

_____

_____

**Eighth Secret**

_____

_____

**Lie I told and to whom**

_____

_____

_____

**Fear**

_____

_____

_____

**Ninth Secret**

_____

_____

**Lie I told and to whom**

_____

_____

_____

**Fear**

_____

_____

**Tenth Secret**

_____

_____

**Lie I told and to whom**

_____

_____

_____

**Fear**

_____

_____

_____

Robert Frost wrote, "The best way out is always through."

One of the best ways to get through your fear is to admit your consequences. Consequences of our choices and actions are difficult to name and to own. They are a sure sign of fallibility and are often inconvenient and painful. They are reality staring you in the face. They force you to reflect upon your distorted thinking. Overcoming denial of consequences is the beginning of a grief process. Listing the disasters and debacles of your life creates a starting point from which you can begin to get a grip on reality. Addiction is a disorder characterized by denial. Addicts lie to, cheat on, and steal from themselves and those they love. There are many times when no one comments on the addict's acting out or the damage the addiction has caused. As a result, it is likely you have overlooked many of the consequences of your substance use. Life consequences often accumulate over time. For an addict, they eventually have so much significance that life itself seems unmanageable. You may find this to be the most difficult exercise to complete in this chapter, but it is also the most useful.

## Exercise 6:   Making a Consequences Inventory

Consider those important social, work-related, family, or recreational activities that you have given up or reduced because of substance use or preoccupation. Include such activities for the entire time you've been using your drug. Next, consider how your drug use made you and others you know feel. Put a check in the box by each of the consequences you have experienced. Put question marks beside the box for each consequence you might have experienced but are not sure. Circle any boxes that contain things you have not experienced but that others have experienced as a result of your using or your behavior.

# Emotional Consequences

❑  Acting against your own values or beliefs

❑  Strong feelings of guilt associated with using

❑  Feelings of shame associated with your behavior

❑  Feelings of isolation or loneliness

❑  Fears of losing your primary relationship

❑  Fears of losing ties with family members or children

❑ Strong feelings of uncertainty for your job, your future

❑ Loss of self-value

❑ Mental-health disorders including depression, anxiety, and traumatic stress

❑ Problematic relationships, affairs, unplanned children, abortion

# Health Consequences

❑ Engaging in drug use despite health problems

❑ Significant weight loss or weight gain

❑ Physical injuries to self or others associated directly with using

❑ Accidental injuries associated with or following drug use

❑ High-risk activities, such as speeding or reckless driving, snowmobiling, off-road vehicle use, mountain climbing, cycling, or boating while under the influence of substances

❑ Sleep disturbances, physical and mental exhaustion

❑ Medical disorders such as headaches, ulcers, high blood pressure, pancreatitis, heart problems, lung problems, malnutrition, bowel problems, sexual problems, infectious diseases such as sinusitis, pneumonia, abscesses, sexually transmitted diseases, HIV and AIDS, hepatitis A, B, or C

❑ Unwanted or unplanned pregnancies

# Family Consequences

❑ Increased tension or increased problems in marriage or primary relationship

❑ Problems with parents or children

❑ Isolation from family-of-origin members

❏ Threatened loss of partner or spouse

❏ Loss of partner or spouse

# Career and Educational Consequences

❏ Change in work habits, dress

❏ Decrease in quality of work

❏ Decrease in productivity

❏ Late to work or appointments, leaving early

❏ Unaccounted-for periods of time away from work

❏ Increased absences or those occurring without timely notification

❏ Loss of credibility, respect at work

❏ Demotion or termination

❏ Frequent job changes or moves

❏ Loss of educational opportunities or work promotions

❏ Poor school performance

# Financial Consequences

❏ Loss of income

❏ Poor investments, high-risk ventures

❏ Gambling on commodities, Internet trading beyond means

❏ Unaccounted-for withdrawals from bank accounts or credit cards

❏ Approximate cost of obtaining your substance, maintaining supply [estimate the actual cost for each of the past five years]

❏ Cost of legal defense for DWIs or other drug-related arrests

# Spiritual Consequences

☐ Emptiness and despair

☐ Disconnection from faith leaders, community of faith, or God of your understanding

☐ Feelings of abandonment by God

☐ Shame about relationship with God

☐ Anger toward God, religious institutions, or people

# Additional Consequences

☐ Loss of interest in hobbies, sports, or other activities

☐ Loss of friendships

☐ Involvement in illegal activities

☐ Shoplifting, stealing, or embezzling money

☐ History of driving-related legal problems, including DWIs, accidents

☐ Legal problems such as arrests, lawsuits, loss of professional licenses

How did life get this way? How did things get so out of hand? It's *denial.* The definition at the start of the chapter says it—a refusal to believe or accept. I refuse to believe I have an addiction or that I continually put myself in harm's way. So far, what have you learned from this chapter? In what ways does the evidence you have written here add to your motivation to change? In what ways will your life be better if you do change? What will be the hardest part about changing?

Facing all the consequences while trying to stop using is often seen as the toughest part of making that change.

# Breaking through Denial and Getting Help

Having done the exercises in this chapter, you might be asking yourself by now,

**Could I be an alcoholic?**

**Could I be an addict?**

The potential for release from any chemical addiction begins with this thought, a thought that, once present, cannot be forgotten. In time, you will find yourself seriously considering the next possibility:

**Perhaps I *am* an addict.**

**Perhaps I *am* addicted to . . .**

This single thought represents a seed of doubt and recognition. Within this seed lies the potential for transformation and the opportunity to discover the true freedom you have been searching for. But even if you are open to the possibility that you are an addict, the reality is that it is very difficult to get sober alone. Fortunately, you don't have to. In the following chapters we will describe in detail, step by step, how you can get help and recover. Here is a brief preview:

1.  Quit floating on the river of Denial, and step onto solid ground. In other words, recognize that you have a problem that is causing you increasing difficulties and that you've been unsuccessful in solving yourself. If you have worked through the exercises in this chapter and see that your behavior is problematic, then you already have a good start. You may still be uncertain about whether you are addicted to some mood-altering drug. Don't beat up on yourself about your ambivalence. Just remember that denial is an integral part of addictive disorders.

2.  Consider the advantage of not going it alone. Most addicts are afraid to trust others, believing that they can depend only on themselves. Recovery is most likely for people who recognize that forces beyond themselves can help them. These forces can include God, nature, and other people. Developing a relationship with a higher power brings a great sense of relief, of realization that you have additional sources of help. Instead of fighting the battle alone, you can "let go and let God." Trusting in a power greater than

yourself combats the depression and sense of helplessness that often results when you finally give up denial and recognize you have a problem that is out of your control.

3. Surround yourself with other recovering people. Until now, your buddies were probably people who, like yourself, enjoyed drinking and drugging. Your relationships with them may have been based on using—hanging out at the bar, partying at people's homes, etc. The conversation, especially if you are male, may have included a lot of bravado, talk about sports and work, but not really revealing yourself. Women tend to open up to their friends more than men, but women addicts often have many secrets to hide (for example, childhood sexual abuse or shame about parenting style) and therefore are also inclined to be emotionally isolated.

A recovering community, such as Alcoholics Anonymous (AA) and other twelve-step programs based on AA, consists of individuals who share the same problem (addiction and how it has made their lives unmanageable) and the same goal—to get sober and remain sober. Unlike your previous social circle, they will not encourage you to drink, but rather to follow the steps of recovery. They are safe to be around. The meetings encourage members to open up about their feelings, and it feels safer to do so because they've been through the same experiences and you know they truly understand you and will not judge or condemn you. Twelve-step meetings are widely available in the United States and other countries, so wherever you travel you can always find members of this community who can give you support and shore up your commitment to recovery should it falter.

Twelve-step meetings are not just social get-togethers. They have a specific purpose—to help the addict recover—and they have a path to do it—the 12 Steps. The steps guide the addict to overcoming denial, trusting in others and a higher power, admitting their past mistakes, making amends to others, continuing to monitor their own behavior, and reaching out to others in need.

Twelve-step meetings are also the place to find a mentor, called a "sponsor," someone who has been in recovery for some time and who can guide you along your journey. We will discuss in later chapters the requirements and role of the mentor. It's very helpful

**Chapter One:** Denial and Other Forms of Brain Trickery | **33**

to choose a sponsor very early in your recovery. Sometimes you may have to try out more than person until you find a good fit, so we suggest you begin by asking someone to be your "temporary sponsor," and see how it works out. The sponsor is person who will monitor you and "tell it like it is," and he or she will also guide you in formally working through the 12 Steps.

As you read the paragraphs above, you might have been feeling a lot of resistance. Addicts often say, "I don't want to sit with a bunch of addicts and hear their sad stories!" or "I'm not going to reveal myself to a group of strangers!" Or, "I'm a pillar of my community—I can't afford to go to an AA meeting where someone might recognize me and spill the beans." Or, "I don't believe in God and I don't want go to a religious meeting. It'll be just a lot of mumbo jumbo."

It is common to feel resistance to going to twelve-step meetings. The stated reasons above usually cover addicts' underlying distrust of other people, fear of letting down their guard and revealing themselves to others, shame about their previous behavior, and lack of knowledge about what really goes on at meetings. The best way to overcome the resistance is to find some "open" AA meetings— those where anyone, not only addicts, can attend, and go to them and just sit and listen. When you're ready to get more involved, go to a "closed" meeting. If someone sees you there, so what? Because only addicts can go to a closed meeting, the person who sees you is also revealing himself or herself to be an addict as well. Read some AA material; you will quickly notice that twelve-step meetings are *not* religious; in fact, mention of any specific religion is against their traditions. Rather, they are *spiritually based*, meaning they believe that help can be gotten from a power greater than oneself, whatever you choose to believe that power to be.

4.  Find a counselor or therapist. As a newcomer, your best bet is to find a professional who is knowledgeable in addictions. He or she can help you assess your need for addiction treatment, and can help you overcome your resistance to group involvement. If you have a slip or relapse, the counselor can work with you on understanding what happened and on putting in place relapse-prevention strategies. Later, when it is time to work on other issues such

as what happened in your childhood, one-on-one therapy can be very helpful. Even later, if your primary relationship has suffered as a result of the addiction, couples' counseling can help rebuild it.

# Being Accountable

Can you think of occasions, during the months and years that you were drinking and drugging, when you were irresponsible? Times when you made promises and didn't keep them? Occasions when you spent money on your addiction that was supposed to be used for family or business expenses? And how about all the times you lied, dissembled, covered up, stretched the truth, and omitted important parts of what had happened? If you are like most addicts, you have a long history of not being accountable to others, coupled with a history of dishonesty in the service of protecting your stash and your ability to continue drinking or drugging. And if you are like most addicts, there were times you felt shame over your behavior, and your self-esteem suffered.

In recovery, it's crucial to reverse this process. Successful recovery demands accountability. You need to practice following through on your commitments. An important part of this is honesty. The founders of AA recognized this a long time ago. This is why the twelve-step program is called a program of "rigorous honesty." Early in recovery, honesty includes telling your partner, counselor, and sponsor about all the drugs you have used, and all the behaviors that you recognized have become compulsive for you. This is not easy, and it may result in unpleasant repercussions. In later chapters, we will discuss the best ways to disclose various addiction secrets. You can also find a detailed guide to disclosure in our book, *Disclosing Secrets: When, To Whom, and How Much to Reveal* (Gentle Path Press, 2002).

Finally: Have you or anyone close you been diagnosed with a serious medical disorder? Most people agree that it helps to have knowledge of your illness. In the past few years, millions of people have researched medical problems on the Internet or read books and magazines in an attempt to become better informed about what's wrong with them. In the next chapter, we will give you some basic information to help you understand the nature of addiction. You are taking an important step in reclaiming your life by the work you do here—welcome!

# CHAPTER TWO: Understanding the Nature of Drug Addiction

**understanding** n. *the power to think, learn, judge*
**nature** n. *the qualities that make something what it is*

If you have been confused about what constitutes addiction to a mood-altering substance, you are not alone. Take comfort in the fact that any confusion you are experiencing is a reflection of the struggle mankind has encountered throughout recorded history. For many centuries, most of the influential voices in Western culture have considered excessive drinking to be a moral and spiritual problem. Those afflicted were believed to lack willpower or to be possessed by some evil influence. Only recently have we come to understand that drug addiction is both a psychological and bio-chemical disorder, not a weakness of character.

Let's start by reviewing the history of drug addiction. Substance-related disorders have been a vexing major public-health problem for most countries since the beginning of recorded history. Drunkenness was a problem in ancient Rome. Opium addiction in China led to the "Opium Wars" in 1839–42 between China and Britain, and in 1856–60 between China and a British-French alliance. Alcoholism in Russia has been a huge problem for many decades. In the United States, the "War on Drugs" that has been waged by the government for the last 25 years is clearly being lost. In 1962, a national survey on substance use concluded that fewer than 4 million Americans had *ever used an illicit drug*; by 1992, a similar survey estimated that approximately 80 million had used an illicit drug at some time in the past. The two surveys support the conclusion that illicit drug use increased 2,000 percent in only three decades!

During this same time, the manifestations of substance dependency changed dramatically. In the early 1960s, the vast majority of patients presenting for alcohol treatment were males addicted only to alcohol. They commonly did not use or abuse any of the other classes of addictive substances, except for nicotine and caffeine, neither of which was generally regarded as addictive at that time. The *Big Book of Alcoholics Anonymous* was first published in 1936, when AA was in its infancy. During the ensuing decades, millions of people in the United States and abroad were able to abstain from drinking alcohol and achieve a level of recovery that they chose to interpret as a "spiritual awakening"—a result of living by the 12 Steps, maintaining a commitment to the fellowship of AA, and asking for the help of God as personally understood. A poignant and unfortunate complication awaited Bill Wilson, one of the primary founders of AA, and many hundreds of thousands in the recovering community. They would die prematurely as a result of lung cancer, emphysema, or heart disease that subsequently was proven to be a direct consequence of nicotine addiction. With the greater understanding of the ill effects of nicotine, many chemical-dependency treatment centers are now smoke free.

The 1960s ushered in a period of idealism and personal freedom, and a climate of permissiveness. As illicit drug use became more prevalent, and indirectly more acceptable, illicit drugs became more available; market dynamics (supply versus demand) resulted in generally lower prices for contraband drugs. During the 1970s and early 1980s, a far wider array of mood-altering street drugs became available, including both illicit and prescription drugs. In the early 1980s, a treatment industry was established which was more or less modeled after the program offered at Hazelden, a treatment center outside of Minneapolis. The "Minnesota model" of treatment was generally regarded as "state of the art." Treatment centers incorporated twelve-step principles and step work, in combination with psychoeducation, group counseling, and other services.

In the early 1980s, professionals who worked at recovery centers began to recognize that the typical patient coming for treatment was far different than before. "Classic alcoholics" were now infrequently seen. The "average" patient was at least a decade younger, had experience with drinking alcohol in high school or within the next few years, and had commonly experimented with illicit substances. By the time life had become unmanageable, patients typically had had significant consequences from the use of two or more substances. Smoking marijuana was very popular as an alternative to getting drunk. Drug histories became more complex. Some combined several drugs while others tended to switch from drug to drug.

Effective treatment programming became much more challenging, and keeping patients together in the meaningful therapeutic groups became far more difficult. Patients were far more diverse, and women were now more comfortable with treatment and came in increasing numbers. This was the heyday of the twenty-eight-day residential programs. Limited evaluation and treatment of other mental disorders was requested by patients or required by licensure regulations.

This historical background may be helpful to you as you reflect upon your own substance-use patterns and associated life problems and consider the prospect of finding the rehabilitation program that's right for you. The point is that substance addiction is a different entity today than it was even fifteen years ago. Patterns of use, the number of different drugs used, and the ritualized patterns that each person creates around drug use have changed significantly. Patients now commonly present with complex disorders that can involve what has been called "dual diagnosis," which means that the patient has some other mental disorder that requires treatment in addition to substance dependency. Other patients have a blend of chemical and behavioral addictions (to gambling, food, sex, work, and risk taking) and may switch from one addiction to another. At the same time that treatment has become more complex, insurance companies have decreased their reimbursement, so that most inpatients no longer are able to stay for twenty-eight days.

Addiction is now understood to be a psychosocial disease that results from disordered chemistry within the body and mind of a genetically susceptible person as the result of using a particular substance over time. In this chapter, we will discuss the nature of addiction, the factors that lead a person to become an addict, and how the multitude of addictive drugs that are now available affect the brain.

# My Love Affair with Drugs

In 1996, Carolyn Knapp, a recovering alcoholic, wrote a book called *Drinking: A Love Story*. Although during her many years of alcoholic drinking she had had several romantic relationships, she realized in retrospect that her most important love affair had been with the bottle. In Exercise 2 in Chapter 1, you began the process of taking a close look at the relationship you have with a substance or several substances. You have considered the ways in which this relationship can take on some of the features of a love object and become at least metaphorically a lover. Like the person you love, you may recall the first time you met your favorite drug; the special names you may be calling it; how meeting it made you feel; how your relationship with the drug resulted in your changing your appearance, hobbies, favorite activities, ability to make friends, and areas of interest; and how the relationship has changed. Like a lover, your drug of choice may have the highest priority in your life. It has been your best friend and lover, a true love affair. Reflect upon how you fell into and perhaps out of "love." You may discover that each of the mood altering substances you have used has its own unique personality and charm. Do you have a number of "lovers," each employed at different settings and occasions, or do you have only one "true love?" You may know some people who have actually referred to their mood-altering substance of choice as "my best friend," or "the one I sleep with to keep me company" for this reason.

Since you have been using this substance, have other people whom you have known for a long time told you that you seem to be a different person? Robert Louis Stevenson wrote *The Strange Case of Dr. Jekyll and Mr. Hyde* in 1886. This little masterpiece is a metaphorical portrayal of addiction in a riveting story that has always intrigued readers. The very names of the hero and antihero have become part of the English language. Dr. Jekyll, a respected scientist, has decided to conduct an experiment upon himself. He begins to use a substance that transforms him into a brutal and savage madman, Mr. Hyde. The scientist keeps a journal of his experiments, carefully noting each element of change and each thought that enters his head. As the experiments progress and as the magical powders cast their spell over him, he loses the ability to separate the potential for good from the impending disaster.

# What Is Addiction?

Substance addiction can be considered as a pathological relationship with a mood-altering drug. The substances may be acquired legally or illegally, and may or may not require a doctor's prescription. They can be swallowed, inhaled, or injected into the body. A few can even be absorbed through the skin. Generally, drugs are abused before addiction sets in. Drug abuse is often termed *misuse* because at this early stage the drug is used by choice and is intentional. What makes it abuse versus recreational use is that it is used in illegal or unsafe situations, or at inappropriate times or places, or in cases where the drug use is harmful to oneself or others. The latest "official" definition of substance dependency, found in the fourth edition of the *Diagnostic and Statistical Manual of Mental Disorders* (DSM-IV) lists seven criteria, at least three of which must be met over a period of several months.

Most of the criteria are psychological rather than physical and can be summarized as three essential features:

1.  Loss of control (compulsive use)

    The DSM-IV describes this as "the substance is often taken in larger amounts or over a longer period than was intended," and "there is a persistent desire or unsuccessful efforts to cut down or control substance use."

    Have there been occasions when you've intended to have only one or two beers at the bar but ended up coming home several hours later after drinking a dozen? Or when you planned on snorting only one line of coke at a party, and next thing you know you've been taking hits all night? Are you an expert at quitting because you've done it a dozen times—but resumed use each time?

2.  Continuation of use despite significant consequences

    This means that "important social, occupational, or recreational activities are given up or reduced because of substance use," and "the substance use is continued despite knowledge of having a persistent or recurrent physical or psychological problem that is likely to have been caused or exacerbated by the substance."

    Have you developed depression or mood swings as a result of your drinking or drugging? Have you gotten into arguments or physical fights you wouldn't have had if you were sober? Has your doctor told you that you need to quit drinking because your blood pressure and uric acid level are too high, your liver enzymes are abnormal, or you've developed gastrointestinal bleeding? Has your smoking resulted in emphysema and lung infections but you are continuing to smoke?

    Is your spouse or partner ready to divorce or leave you because of your drug use? Has your lying and covering up affected your relationship with your partner? Are your children frequently disappointed because your drinking or drug use caused you to miss a ball game or other promised activity? Have you narrowed your circle of friends to those who drink or drug with you or given up friends all together? Have you lost your job because you came to work too late one time too many—or because you flunked a urine drug test? Have you been arrested for driving while intoxicated? Have you gotten into a car accident because you were drinking or drugging?

3. Preoccupation or obsession

This means that "a great deal of time is spent in activities necessary to obtain the substance, use the substance or figure out how much you can use to "prove" you are not addicted, or recover from its effects."

Do you spend time at work planning on how to get your next drug? Have you missed work because of hangovers? Have you missed your child's birthday party because you were too busy drinking or drugging?

## Exercise 1:   Applying the Criteria to My Own Drug Use

Below each of the two criteria listed below, write down examples from your own past:

1. Loss of control (compulsive use)

 

 

2. Continuation of use despite adverse consequences

 

 

 

## Exercise 2:   Preoccupation or Obsession

In this exercise, take a few minutes to close your eyes and think about your drug of choice. Then answer the following questions. If your period of heaviest use was more than six months ago, then change the time frame of the question to that period of time.

In the past six months, on average, how many times a day do you believe you thought about using your substance?

 

 

Can you recall what times of day you experienced a desire to use this substance?

 

 

What kinds of activities were associated with your efforts to obtain it or get to a place where you know it would be found?

_____

_____

During the past six months, about how much time each week did you spend protecting your supply [such as hiding or stockpiling] and obtaining your drug of choice?

_____

_____

What memories came to mind? What experiences? Get these down on paper, too.

_____

_____

In addition to the three categories of behavior problems, dependence to some drugs—but not all—causes physiological dependence. When these drugs are used repeatedly, the body makes chemical adjustments to allow the person to continue to function despite the presence of large amounts of the drug in his body. This is why a heavy drinker may be walking around with a blood alcohol level of 0.3 (which is three times the legal limit, or more, in many states), whereas a nondrinker who imbibes enough to raise the blood level to 0.3 is likely to be comatose. The drinker has become _tolerant_ to the effects of alcohol, but at a high cost; when it is suddenly stopped, the drinker will experience a physiological rebound called _withdrawal_. Tolerance and withdrawal go together.

_Tolerance_ is defined in the DSM-IV as "a need for markedly increased amounts of the substance to achieve intoxication or desired effect," along with "markedly diminished effect with continued use of the same amount of the substance."

Have you ever heard some party-goer described as having a "wooden leg" with regard to his drinking? That means he can drink a very large amount without developing slurred speech, loss of balance, or passing out— usual effects of consuming a lot of alcohol. This person, as a result of his prior heavy drinking, has developed tolerance to alcohol. What about the heroin addict who dies suddenly after taking a hit? What has happened is that, although this person has already developed tolerance to the respiratory depressant effect of the usual heroin dose, he has just unknowingly injected a much larger amount of the drug, which has then stopped his breathing.

*Withdrawal* is manifested by characteristic physical effects the person experiences when stopping the drug, which can be relieved by taking either more of the same drug or a closely related substance. Some drugs, like cocaine, a central nervous system stimulant, do not have significant physical withdrawal symptoms in the same way that heroin or alcohol do. Yet, the cocaine addict will tell you that the craving is intense and the emotional withdrawal is hell. Because we now know that emotions change neuro-chemistry in the brain, too, it is easier to see how cocaine's emotional withdrawal also feels bad.

The best-known withdrawal syndromes are those experienced by alcoholics and narcotic addicts who quit cold turkey (or who unexpectedly find themselves separated from their supply). Alcohol withdrawal symptoms include sweating, rapid pulse, hand tremor, insomnia, nausea or vomiting, agitation, anxiety, grand mal seizures, and hallucinations.

*Alcohol withdrawal can be fatal.* The full-blown withdrawal syndrome is rarely seen these days, because it can be avoided with a medically supervised tapering schedule of a benzodiazepine or barbiturate. You can see what it was like before these drugs became available by watching some old movies, such as *Lost Weekend*, about an alcoholic who was detoxed by being placed in a padded room for several days, period. If you are a heavy drinker and want to stop, you should see a physician who can help you detox by admin-istering medication so that you don't have a seizure or some other physi-ological consequence from withdrawal from the drug.

Symptoms from narcotic withdrawal include nausea and vomiting, muscle aches, tearing of the eyes, a runny nose, goose bumps, increased sweating, diarrhea, yawning, fever, and insomnia. These symptoms may be very unpleasant but are not dangerous.

For a person to be addicted to a drug, it's not necessary that they expe-rience withdrawal symptoms if they stop suddenly. We mentioned cocaine earlier. Several other important drugs of abuse do *not* have a specific with-drawal syndrome. These include marijuana, hallucinogens (LSD, mush-rooms), inhalants, and phencyclidine (PCP).

## Exercise 3: Have You Developed Tolerance?

In Chapter One, you wrote out a history of your drug use. Now, to the best of your recollection, write how much of your drug of choice you would use within a twelve- or a twenty-four-hour period of time, which-ever seems most appropriate. Note also any other substances you would use at the same time, or after, to "come down" or to counteract the effects of using. Consider the quantity of use now, three months ago, six months ago, one year ago, and five years ago. Use the following table to help organize your work:

| Period of time | Amount used in a 24-hour period | Other substances used |
|---|---|---|
| Now | | |
| Three months ago | | |
| Six months ago | | |
| One year ago | | |
| Five years ago | | |

Another important characteristic of addiction is that when the drug is stopped, the user may develop a *craving*, or hunger, to use it, which is a persistent desire despite efforts to cut down or stop. Craving is of course worsened when there are physical withdrawal symptoms that you know can be alleviated by using the drug, but even drugs that don't have well-defined withdrawal symptoms can produce intense cravings; cocaine is the best-known example. An important aspect of remaining sober is to learn how to deal with cravings without using. More about that in Chapter 11.

## Exercise 4: Recognition of Drug Hunger (Desire to Use, Craving)

Recall times when you have chosen not to use your substance of choice for days or weeks. What made you decide to return to using? Did you experience any internal changes such as flu-like symptoms or irritability? Did certain people seem to get on your nerves? What situations, which of your friends, seem to be associated with your return to using or drinking? Are there certain places, times of day, times of year, events (such as birthdays, visits to parents, or holidays) that trigger your use?

What moods are associated with the desire to use? On what occasions have you used drugs to solve problems or get back at people who bother you?

This wanting is based upon a mixture of likes and dislikes, attractions and aversions, preferences and judgments about this substance that we have stored in our memory. This is the same type of process your brain uses to store memory of a person you know and love and wish to see once again.

# Why Do Some People Develop Addictions while Others Do Not?

During the Vietnam War, thousands of Americans were uprooted from their usual life and shipped (often involuntarily) to a dangerous environment, where death was often just around the corner, where enemy and friend were often indistinguishable—and where mood-altering drugs were cheap and widely available. Not surprisingly, drug abuse was widespread among the soldiers. Physicians in the United States were convinced that an enormous need for addiction treatment would follow the return home of the soldiers. Surprisingly, this did not happen. Instead, most drug-using soldiers spontaneously stopped using when they returned home, and only a small minority required treatment. Clearly, addiction is not just a matter of repeated exposure to a drug!

We believe that many, if not most people in the world are susceptible to developing a substance-related addiction under some specific set of conditions. The basic clinical formula that results in the development of substance addiction can be expressed in this way:

> The right person [one with genetic predisposition] + right substance [the one that produces a desirable change in mood and perception, at least initially] + factors of gender, age, and ethnicity + vulnerable time in life during which change is desired + right setting/environment = addiction to that substance

The interaction of all of these factors creates addiction. Let's review each one:

1. Physical factors: brain chemistry, genetic predisposition

   Over the past several million years of evolution, animals have taken divergent paths, but all reptiles, birds, and mammals have retained the specialized centers in the central nervous system that reinforced basic drives and motivations. These specialized centers retained the established specific neurochemical rewards for behavior that had proven useful for survival and procreation. These organized common reward centers in the brain receive signals from millions of individual brain cells that are involved in other functions of consciousness, such as sensing objects in the environment and movement of the body. They have remained part of the human brain through its evolution to the present. When we engage in behaviors that are successful in performing actions that feed, shelter, comfort, or protect our body and mind, stimulation of the *pleasure center* of the human brain produces the reward we experience as gratification or appeasement. To date, more than forty brain chemicals are known that function as neurotransmitters. Some are excitatory, that is, they increase brain activity; others are inhibitory. Some of the most well-studied neurotransmitters are dopamine, epinephrine, norepinephrine, serotonin, gamma-aminobutyric acid (GABA), and glutamate. When neurotransmitters are released, the person experiences a feeling of pleasure (reward) for certain behaviors, or a feeling of pain, anxiety, or fear (aversion) that serves as motivation to not repeat the behavior in the future.

When these neurotransmitters stimulate the pleasure center, the neurons in this center put out their own electrical and chemical signals that communicate with the rest of the central nervous system.

*Mood-altering substances* also produce stimulation of the reward system. Different classes of drugs produce neurobiochemical pathway responses through various types of alterations to one or more of the neurotransmitter systems. For example,

- Alcohol and benzodiazepines (such as Valium, Librium, etc.) produce sedative effects through the GABA system.

- Cocaine blocks the reuptake of dopamine by brain cells (and its subsequent inactivation), thereby increasing the level of brain dopamine. Dopamine stimulates the pleasure/reward system in the brain. Amphetamines and other stimulants behave similarly. All of these produce increased arousal.

- Opioids (narcotics) have pre-existing receptors in the brain (and other parts of the body). When those receptors are activated, they send signals that reduce pain and also have a sedative effect.

The biochemical details of how each mood-altering substance works are just being defined in research laboratories around the world. Scientists do know that no matter what pathways are involved along the way, all mood-altering substances eventually stimulate the reward system. Robert DuPont, in his book, *The Selfish Brain*, explains it very clearly:

> When the brain's reward or pleasure centers are stimulated, the brain sends out powerful signals to repeat the pleasure producing behaviors. With respect to aggression, fear feeding [including addictive substances], and sexuality the brain is selfish. It simply wants what it wants right

now. The brain directs the person to relieve distress and to promote pleasure. Automatic brain mechanisms do not consider other people's feelings or needs or know the importance of delayed gratification. That is why I call this basic pleasure/pain organ the selfish brain (p. 3).

When someone ingests, inhales, or injects a mood-altering drug, the molecules of the drug bind with receptors in the brain, producing the neurotransmitters we discussed earlier. But drugs coming into the brain are not the only way to stimulate it. Mood-altering behaviors such as gambling, sex, or risk taking can cause the production of the brain's own chemicals, which have the same reinforcing effect. For example, we now know that the brain can produce its own opiate (narcotic)-like chemicals, called *endorphins* and *enkephalins*, which bind to the same receptors as do morphine, heroin, and other narcotics, and which result in the same good feelings. The bottom line is that *all addictions trigger the same underlying brain-reward mechanisms*. This is true whether the addiction is to a drug or a behavior. This scientifically supported disease concept of addiction means that the addict is not simply addicted to a specific drug but that he or she is addicted to brain-rewarding chemicals in general.

Despite the fact that all of us have the same basic brain chemistry, some people are more vulnerable to addiction than others because of their genetic makeup. Among animals, different strains of rats have been bred to have unusually high, or extremely low, predilection for morphine, cocaine, and alcohol. In humans, studies have shown that children of alcoholic parents have a three- to fourfold increased likelihood of becoming alcoholics themselves than do children of nonalcoholics (Schuckit, 1987). This is not just due to their environment: Children of alcoholics who were adopted and raised in nonalcoholic families still had the increased risk of becoming alcoholics. Dr. Mark Schuckit, working with young adult sons of alcoholics, found that, even though they had had very little exposure to alcohol, they were able to drink larger amounts than sons of nonalcoholics before they experienced any mood alteration or decreased functioning. These young men were likely, therefore, to have less motivation to stop after only a few drinks.

The genetics of addiction to drugs other than alcohol have not been as well studied, but, with the rapidly growing information on brain chemistry, it is clear that addiction of all types is biologically influenced. Therefore, it is very likely that genetic factors influence the risk of all addictions. In the next exercise is a family tree of a family with many addicts over the years.

As you can see, many people throughout the generations probably contributed to the man's predisposition toward addiction.

## Exercise 5:   Drawing a Family Tree

Getting a picture of how addiction has been present in your family over generations can help you see how you might have been given the predisposition toward addiction by the genes passed on in your family. Draw your family tree. Identify all the addicts that you know about in your family. If you aren't sure, call someone in the family, or several folks, and ask who was an addict. The history can be any type of addiction, not just alcohol or drug addiction. Also identify other conditions that might lead someone to use drugs, such as medical disorders like bipolar disease or attention deficit disorder/attention deficit hyperactivity disorder (ADD/ADHD). Look back and see what genetic pool you stepped out of. If you are the first to become addicted in your family, what are the reasons to make yourself the last? If you are the fiftieth, what are the reasons to be the last?

# Family Tree

Let's pretend this is your family, that you are male with a cocaine and alcohol addiction. Let's also say that your grandfather on your Dad's side, your Dad and your sister all are addicted to alcohol and your sister is addicted to cocaine and has a gambling problem. Your genogram might look like this:

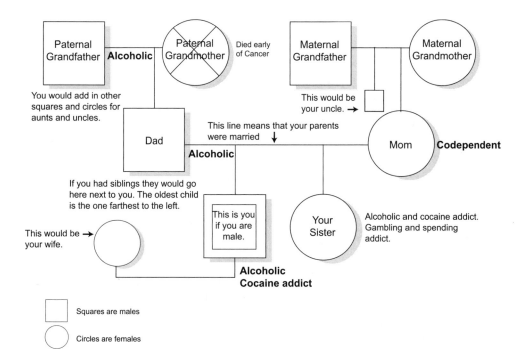

Paternal Grandfather — **Alcoholic**

Paternal Grandmother — Died early of Cancer

Maternal Grandfather

Maternal Grandmother

You would add in other squares and circles for aunts and uncles.

This would be your uncle. →

Dad — **Alcoholic**

This line means that your parents were married ↓

Mom — **Codependent**

If you had siblings they would go here next to you. The oldest child is the one farthest to the left.

This would be → your wife.

This is you if you are male.

Your Sister — Alcoholic and cocaine addict. Gambling and spending addict.

**Alcoholic Cocaine addict**

☐ Squares are males

○ Circles are females

---

**Your Family Tree**

---

2.  Psychological factors: A person's vulnerability is related to one's family of origin and current stresses.

    Scratch any addict and you are likely to find below the surface some underlying psychological vulnerabilities, some pain due to perceived or real childhood experiences, which lead to a desire to escape one's problems through immersion in some pleasure-producing drug or experience. In a study of more than 1,000 sex addicts (many of whom were also chemically addicted), Patrick Carnes (1991) learned that some 81 percent had been sexually abused, 72 percent were physically abused, and 97 percent had been emotionally abused. This is a dismal picture! And it is true not only of sex addicts. A startlingly large percentage of women alcoholics were sexually abused in childhood. Many future drug addicts were raised in homes where one or more adults was chemically dependent. Even if the addicted parent was not physically (or sexually) abusive, he was not very available to the child, as the addiction had top priority. Or perhaps a family member was ill and received the bulk of the attention, or maybe a parent was very involved in their career and rarely home. No matter what the circumstance, the result may have been that the child felt a lack of nurturing, came to believe that he was not sufficiently loved because he was unlovable, felt responsible for the family's happiness, and so on. Some such children become family heroes, whereas others escape into a private world of fantasy. Still others draw attention to themselves because of their bad behavior.

As they grow up, children from dysfunctional families develop a set of *faulty core beliefs*, which may include:

- I am basically a bad, unworthy person.
- No one will love me as I am.
- My needs are never going to be met if I have to depend on others.
- Alcohol (or other drug of choice) is my most important need.

They may look good on the outside, but on the inside they have low self-esteem and a basic distrust of others. They have a core of shame—they feel bad about who they are. Sooner or later, many of them find that some drug or behavior fills the hole inside them and dulls the pain. At first the drug is very effective, but in many cases it eventually begins to control the person, the pleasure or relief diminishes, and the addict has to keep using just to feel normal.

Figure 2.1, later in the chapter, shows how the process keeps feeding itself. The person's faulty belief system leads to using psychological defenses instead of seeing the truth. These are forms of *impaired thinking*. These include:

- Denial: "I don't have a problem," "I don't need anyone."

- Minimization: "It's no big deal if I missed my anniversary dinner with my wife, she doesn't really love me anyway."

- Intellectualization: "The only way I can survive is to be in control." Otherwise something bad will happen. It is almost as if you have a voice in your head that belongs to your addict. That voice reasons that life is better because of how your drug has supposedly helped you in the past. That voice will defend your use in the past and justify your right to decide whether you can use in the future. It will suppress your emotions and your ability to listen to any negative opinions you might hear about your drug use or its effects on you.

- Rationalization. "It's my boss's fault I keep drinking—anyone would in my position." These defenses impair your thinking and prevent you from recognizing the negative consequences of your drinking or drugging. But they do not prevent you from feeling the shame and worthlessness that result from your underlying belief system.

The inability to tolerate those emotions connected to the belief system is a trigger that invites the desire to use in hopes of making the feeling go away. Over time, this is so automatic that you can be triggered by the emotions connected to the underlying belief system and not even recognize it has happened—what you can recognize is that you have started obsessing about how you can be released from the bad feelings.

Seeking release from these bad feelings, the addict escapes into *preoccupation* or *obsession,* one of the key features of addiction. Sometimes the preoccupation is related to the obsessive thoughts about what is happening that is contributing to the faulty core beliefs. Sometimes it is about obtaining the drug or thinking about how it feels to use the drug. We often call this *euphoric recall.*

---

Some people who are extremely depressed also obsess about staying depressed. They become so accustomed to being depressed that it is almost frightening to think about being without the misery. This might sound weird to someone who loves the euphoric high, but someone who experiences living in this "black hole" fears that he or she could not survive outside this "black hole." Consequently, these people spend time depriving themselves of anything that might help them make a movement beyond this terrible depressing state. Self-statements and their own preoccupation are connected to this state of mind. Their drug use, while in the beginning might have been an effort to not feel so bad, over time has resulted in seeking a dysphoric state of mind. This deprivation cycle is common in people with some forms of eating disorders. It is also common in some drug addicts.

---

## Exercise 6:  Preoccupation

Make a list of situations you can recall when you have been preoccupied or obsessed by thoughts about yourself and your faulty core beliefs or of your drug of choice or plans for using it:

_____

_____

_____

_____

_____

_____

_____

Being preoccupied and obsessing are really the first part of *ritualization*. A ritual is nothing more than a set of behaviors and thoughts that, when repeated over and over, become second nature and work almost automatically. Think about when you began to use on a regular basis. At times, you might have had this persistent feeling and you were not exactly sure how the drug use got started. It was almost as if you were in a hypnotic trance. Then you might have had a sense of condensed or lost time, then a sense of not knowing exactly where you were or what had just happened, although this feeling lasted only seconds. Then there was a sense of re-orientation. All of this is like seizure activity but also like going in and out of a hypnotic trance. A trance is the process of taking your focus from the general to the specific, gradually so narrowing your focus that at the time you are also suggestible to other things. This is why people make poor decisions even before they use their drug of choice—because the brain already begins to respond chemically when it is stimulated by the memory of drug use as part of the ritual.

## Exercise 7:   Your Drug Ritual

Write out in detail your ritual for using your favorite drug. Do you use it the same way each time? Notice the effect on you just from thinking about this! Caution: It may be wise to have another recovering person with you in the room when you do this exercise, because it may result in a strong desire to use.

_____

_____

_____

_____

_____

_____

_____

_____

By the time the user completes his ritual, he is already in an altered state, anxious to move ahead to *action!* Now is the time to proceed with "acting out," which means using the drug or carrying out the addictive behavior. You no longer are aware of the self-defeating and self-destructive nature of your activity—you are totally focused on getting the reward. Unfortunately, once you have finished using, reality sets in again, and with it comes despair and self-loathing. Yet, it is not even the craving, the desire to use again, that is the cause of your anger and fear, but rather judging yourself harshly because of your lack of willpower, your weakness, or your immorality. You tell yourself that the addiction is the result of your evil desires, your selfish cravings, your helplessness, and your laziness—further proof that you are bad and unworthy. It's too painful to remain in this state for long, but soon enough your impaired thinking comes to your rescue.

**Figure 2.1**

# The Addictive System

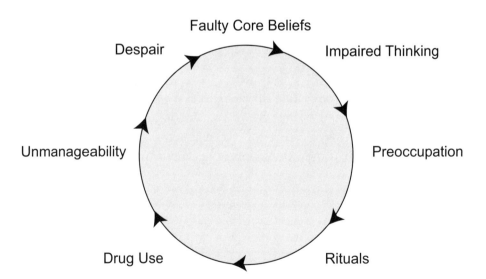

You make excuses, blame others, and minimize the damage. Once again you're caught in the addictive cycle (see Figure 2.1).

3. Environmental factors: availability of the drug, encouragement from others

   If a drug is unavailable, even the most genetically and psychologically vulnerable person is unlikely to become addicted to that drug. This is only common sense! When cocaine was available only as an expensive powder, cocaine addicts were few and generally well-off financially. But when rocks of crack cocaine for smoking became available on the streets in large quantities and low cost, a cocaine epidemic suddenly spread like wildfire. The cause of the current epidemic is the increased availability and affordability of the drug. The same is true of alcohol and nicotine, the two most prevalent addictive drugs. These drugs also have the advantage of being legal, which means that they are openly sold in every corner drug store and grocery store.

   Encouragement from others also promotes addiction. When you were trying to stay away from alcohol, did any of your friends ever tell you at a party, "Oh, come on—just have one drink. It will relax you?" Or, having decided to no longer smoke pot, have you been tempted when seeing a group of your friends smoking, laughing, and gobbling down munchies? This is why it is important in recovery to change your social circle and avoid your drug-using friends. Then there's the encouragement provided by advertisements and TV and radio commercials. Until they were banned from radio and TV, commercials for cigarettes were ubiquitous. You could hardly turn on your television set without seeing a group of sexy, attractive, young people smoking or chugging down a beer. The message was, you can be sexy and popular if you smoke. Remember those commercials, targeted at women, that showed an attractive young woman in an evening gown smoking while a good-looking man attended to her? The message was, you can be slender and sophisticated if you smoke, as well as be attractive to desirable men. The recognition that people are vulnerable to such advertising has led to laws that have banned much of it.

## Exercise 8:   Your Environmental influences

Write a list of examples of circumstances when other people or outside influences resulted in your drinking or drugging.

_____

Figure 2.1 summarizes the way all the factors we have just discussed interact to bring about drug use. Addicts typically go round and round in this circle, each factor reinforcing the others and ending up in a repetitive cycle of drug use.

And it can get even more complicated! As we said above, most drug addicts these days use more than one drug. And in addition, many drug addicts are simultaneously also addicted to behaviors, such as gambling, sex, work, risk taking, or eating disorders. In addition, many addicts also have psychological disorders. In the next chapter we will describe what happens when a person has a combination of addictions and mental disorders.

## References

Carnes, P. (1991). *Don't Call It Love.* New York: Bantam Books, p. 109.

Diagnostic and Statistical Manual of Mental Disorders, 4th ed. (DSM-IV). Washington, D.C: American Psychiatric Press, pp. 176–82.

DuPont, R. (1997). *The Selfish Brain: Learning From Addiction.* Washington, D.C.: American Psychiatric Press, pp. 101–124.

Knapp, C. (1996). *Drinking: A Love Story.* New York: Dial Press.

Schuckit, MA (1984a). Ethanol-induced changes in body sway in men at high alcoholism risk. *Archives of General Psychiatry* 42:375–379;

Schuckit, MA (1984b). Subjective responses to alcohol in sons of alcoholics and controls. *Archives of General Psychiatry* 41:879–884.

Schuckit , MA. (1987). Biological vulnerability to alcoholism. *Journal of Consulting and Clinical Psychology* 55:301–309.

# CHAPTER THREE: Double Your Pleasure, Double Your Trouble:

## *Combining Drugs and Behaviors*

**double** adj. *twice as much*
**trouble** v. *to cause mental agitation, pain or discomfort*

When the *Big Book* was published in 1936, it addressed only alcohol addiction, because virtually all of its members were addicted only to alcohol. (To be more accurate, we would have to say they were addicted to alcohol and nicotine, but in 1936 no one thought tobacco/nicotine was a problem.) Today, in contrast, most addicts believe in "polypharmacy," which means combining drugs in an attempt to obtain more pleasure or a better outcome. The most common example is combining alcohol and cigarettes. There is a strong correlation between smoking and drinking. This means that a much larger percentage of alcoholics smoke than do nonalcoholics. Another popular combination is cocaine and alcohol. In one study of cocaine addicts, alcoholism was the most frequently diagnosed coexisting psychiatric disorder, and alcoholism was associated with more severe cocaine dependence (Carroll et al., 1993). The alcohol is used to combat the anxiety and sleep disruption caused by cocaine. In addition, alcohol and cocaine in the body combine to produce cocaethylene, a substance that may enhance and prolong cocaine euphoria.

Whereas cocaine and alcohol have opposite effects on the body, some drugs have very similar effects and are used to substitute for one another or enhance the effects of the preferred drug. For example, benzodiazepines work like alcohol, so that combining alcohol and benzos is like having more to drink. In someone who's experiencing withdrawal symptoms from having suddenly stopped alcohol, benzodiazepines can prevent and relieve withdrawal. In the same way, heroin addicts use other narcotics, such as the prescription drugs hydrocodone and oxycodone, to prevent withdrawal if they are unable to obtain heroin.

About 70 percent of cocaine addicts are also sexually compulsive. Unfortunately for male cocaine addicts on a binge, men can perform sexually only a limited number of times per day. To enhance their sexual performance, some men are now adding the anti–erectile dysfunction drug Viagra (sildanefil) to the mix, using it along with cocaine to prolong their cocaine-sex binge. Viagra has been mixed with ecstasy (called sextasy), poppers, methamphetamine, and other types of speed to enhance erectile ability. Caution: Do not try this—there is a high risk of a heart attack. Less lethal, but certainly a painful condition for ecstasy users, are severe head-aches; other male drug users report incidents of prolonged, painful erections (priapism) that for some have to be surgically corrected. Talk about giving yourself a reason to avoid future sexual dysfunction!

These are just a few examples of creative chemistry among drug addicts. Unfortunately, combining drugs can also cause combined health risks. In Chapter 5 we will describe how different drugs damage the body. In brief, alcohol and cigarettes are probably the two most dangerous drugs around in terms of their health consequences. Alcohol can cause high blood pressure, liver damage, gastrointestinal bleeding, gout, heart damage, and automobile and pedestrian accidents. Cigarettes can cause cancer of the lung, throat, and bladder. Smoking also causes emphysema, heart disease, strokes, and narrow-ing of the blood vessels in the legs. When both drugs are used together, the damage to the body is increased.

The same is true for alcohol and cocaine. Cocaine constricts blood vessels, including those in the brain and heart. It can cause strokes, heart attacks, and sudden death. Combine it with alcohol, and you are likely to experience the damage that both drugs can produce.

In addition to the physical consequences, combining drugs can make it harder to recover. When the two drugs are part of the same ritual, it is very hard to stop one if you continue the other. Say you have decided to stop drinking any form of alcohol. If your ritual included smoking a cigarette as you drank a beer, you are likely to feel an intense desire for a beer the minute you light up a cigarette. The only solution is to stop *both* smoking and drinking. This is, of course, harder than stopping only one drug. The same is true when your concurrent addiction is a behavior rather than a drug. This will be discussed in the next section.

# Exercise 1:   Your Use of More than One Drug

Think about other drugs you have used in addition to your drug of choice. Write a list of these drugs and how they interacted with your drug of choice.

1. _____

_____

2. _____

_____

3. _____

_____

4. _____

_____

5. _____

_____

6. _____

_____

7. _____

_____

8. _____

_____

9. _____

_____

10. _____

_____

# Complicating Matters—Combing Drugs with Behaviors

We have already mentioned the combined use of cocaine with sexual behaviors. This is one of the most common and potentially dangerous combinations because, over time, the behaviors become pair-bonded. In other words, when you do one behavior, it stimulates the brain chemistry for the other and makes you crave. So if you give up cocaine and addictive sex, but want to return to healthy sex, you will find it difficult to get beyond that craving for the cocaine when you first begin to engage in healthy sex. This can be very troublesome for people, and the accompanying anxiety contributes to sexual dysfunction problems and can trigger a relapse as well.

This is true of all stimulants (cocaine, amphetamines). They make people feel less inhibited and they heighten the interest in sex. Not only is it harder to give up the drug and get the behavior under control, but combining the drug with the sexual behavior increases the chances that you will put yourself and/or others in harm's way. You just don't make good decisions when your brain is laced with or drowning in the effects of the drug. You are likely to forget to use condoms to prevent pregnancy and sexually transmitted diseases (STDs), and you may continue the behavior to the point of self-injury. If you combine these drugs with sexual behavior at a club, you may find yourself in a dangerous situation where you may be robbed, beaten, or killed. With HIV and all the other sexually transmitted viruses and diseases, combining drugs with behavior is a huge problem.

There are many ways people combine sexual behavior (which creates its own mood-altering drug in your head) with drugs. Smoking many cigarettes while masturbating can invite a nicotine overdose, which is dangerous for your heart. Some people have died when they combined experimental or addictive sex with too many stimulants, narcotics, depressants, or hallucinogens.

Of course, casinos have figured out that alcohol helps you make dumb bets and that nicotine keeps you stimulated so you will stay longer. There is no shortage of cheap drinks, and you can smoke until the sun comes up while gambling. In the end, the casinos win much more often than the gambler. If you are a compulsive gambler, chances are high that you will also be a compulsive smoker and that you will abuse alcohol, if you are not dependent on it, because smoking and drinking become part of the ritual. That means you have three addictions to conquer instead of one.

Diet products have promised such wonders to food addicts, but many of those products are actually addictive stimulants. If your body is already compromised by extra weight or not enough nutrition, the added stress of a drug addiction makes it harder to manage everyday activities. This stress becomes a trigger, and you have a vicious addiction cycle.

If you work compulsively, you have already discovered many ways to alter your mood in hopes of making you more creative, to give you more energy, or to help you cope with stress. Eventually the costs of combining the behavior with a drug will come back to haunt you. What was the solution becomes the problem. In the end, combining drug use with behavior that becomes an addictive ritual makes stopping either the drug or the behavioral addiction more difficult.

## Exercise 2:   Ways in Which I Combine Drugs and Behaviors

Not everyone combines drugs with behaviors in their addiction; occasionally they just experiment or discover something by accident. In this exercise, really examine your own drug use and how certain behaviors are part of your ritual. List all drugs you use and the behaviors you engage in during drug use. If you are aware that they are a part of your addiction or that the behavior is the primary addiction and the drug addiction is secondary, make a note of that.

| Drug | Behavior | Note |
|------|----------|------|
|      |          |      |
|      |          |      |
|      |          |      |
|      |          |      |
|      |          |      |
|      |          |      |
|      |          |      |
|      |          |      |
|      |          |      |
|      |          |      |

# Further Complications—Other Disorders that Drug Use Temporarily Soothes

In Chapter 2 we discussed several reasons why some people are vulnerable to drug abuse—their genetic makeup, childhood issues, life stresses, and outside influences. There's one other vulnerability that bears mention: physical or psychiatric disorders. Some psychiatric disorders affect people's judgment so that they are likely to do anything that feels good, including using and abusing alcohol and other drugs. This is particularly true for people with antisocial personality disorder and the manic phase of bipolar illness (or manic-depressive illness). In fact, bipolar disorder is the most common condition seen today in people who have a "dual diagnosis" (addiction plus a psychiatric or physical disorder).

In other cases, however, addicts use alcohol and drugs in an attempt to self-medicate the problems their illness has caused. In such cases, their drug of choice is often one that indeed improves the specific problem (at least initially!). For example,

- _Bipolar Disorder_—On the upswing, patients are likely to abuse *any* mood-altering drug or behavior, including alcohol, narcotics, cocaine, and sex.

- _Psychosis_—When a person becomes disconnected from reality, for example a schizophrenic who is hallucinating, he may seek to escape his fearful inner world by excessive use of alcohol or other drugs.

- _Anxiety disorders_—Alcohol and benzodiazepines sedate and thereby relieve anxiety.

- _Depression_—Mood elevators such as cocaine can improve one's mood.

- _Attention deficit hyperactivity disorder (ADHD)_—Mood elevators such as Ritalin paradoxically calm people with ADHD, which is why it is often prescribed for people with this disorder, especially children.

- _Social phobia_—Fear of being in social situations can be somewhat alleviated by alcohol, which is disinhibiting; it makes people less concerned about their behavior.

- *Insomnia*—Many people use alcohol to help induce sleep. Unfortunately, after a while, it no longer works. The same is true for benzodiazepines (whether prescribed or not).

- *Chronic pain*—Opioids (narcotics) are being increasingly prescribed for all types of chronic pain, usually under strict guidelines and careful medical follow-up. But many people with a pain problem obtain narcotics on the street and use them in growing amounts for their pain.

- *Post-traumatic stress disorder (PTSD,) schizoaffective disorder, and psychosis*— These disorders all create a great deal of anxiety, which sufferers sometimes try to escape by using drugs.

When a drug addict or alcoholic requests treatment, all qualified addiction medicine specialists and treatment centers do an initial assessment for the presence of a dual diagnosis. If present, then both disorders must be treated.

## Exercise 3: My Use of Mood-altering Drugs to Manage Physical or Psychological Conditions

Did your drug use begin as a way to manage another condition? This exercise will help you recognize if you also need to address some other problems in addition to your drug abuse or dependency. Review the list above. In the space provided below indicate all the conditions that you might have tried to solve with your drug use. If you see a pattern but you have yet to consult a doctor about this, now is a good time to do so. There are excellent and safe medications today that can help stabilize these conditions. And most insurance companies will pay for care of these disorders far longer than they will pay for your addiction treatment.

_____

_____

_____

_____

_____

_____

# Your Addictive Cycle

At the end of Chapter 2 we showed you the addictive cycle in which addicts get caught. It is now time for you to identify how your own addictive cycle works. Below is a graphic representation of the addictive cycle with space for examples from your own life. You may have so much information that you need more room. Some people use a large piece of paper and diagram their own addictive system. Take each component, faulty core beliefs, impaired thinking, preoccupation, ritualization, drug use, despair, and unmanageability and begin to map out your addiction. It is important to review this with your therapist, sponsor, or others in your support system.

**Figure 3.1**

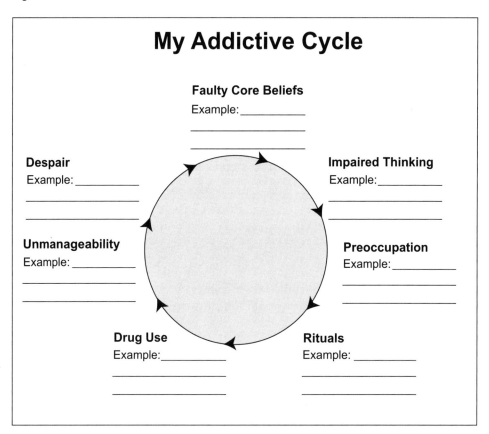

Freedom from the recurring desire to return to your substance use requires a shift in thinking and perception. You can use that desire instead to search for an end to intrusive thoughts, for freedom from craving, for growth along spiritual lines, to overcome the desire to use again, and to heal the shame that prevents you from believing there is hope. You must come to appreciate that desire is not really the problem. Having the desire to use is not right or wrong. It is your attachment to the drug identified with that particular desire that is the cause of your pain and suffering. In order to give up this attachment, you must want to become the male or female hero who overcomes adversity rather than the victim of fate. You must admit that you need help from others in order to choose the right path to follow. If you are addicted, you must find out and do something about it. You must find the strength and will to experience the living truth about your attachment to this substance. Your pathologic attachment to this substance does not mean you are destined to be addicted to every other substance in the world. You are now about to embark on a journey. The next few chapters will show you how to start on the path to recovery.

## References

Carroll KM, Rounsaville JB, & Bryant KJ. 1993. Alcoholism in treatment-seeking cocaine abusers: Clinical and prognostic significance. *Journal of Studies of Alcohol* 54:199–208.

*Diagnostic and Statistical Manual of Mental Disorders, 4th ed.* 1994, (DSM-IV). Washington, D.C: American Psychiatric Press.

# CHAPTER FOUR: Embrace the Process

**embrace** v. *to take up or adopt eagerly or seriously*
**process** n. *a continuing development involving many changes*

A new member of an addiction treatment group once asked how you get through this initial, uncomfortable stage of recovery. Another man with several years' experience in recovery, Dan, shared that when he was sent to treatment he thought all of the counselors and staff were crazy and that he was the only sane one there. Dan related how he put up every possible road block during that first phase of his treatment, trying to convince everyone that his problem was not all that bad and that being in treatment was not the answer. But as he began to examine all the ways that his drug-using behavior went against what he wanted to believe about himself, and how his drug use was inconsistent with his values, he realized that his life had become unmanageable and that he was indeed powerless over his addiction. Dan recounted the many ways his life had spun out of control and how much he had hurt his wife, co-workers, and most of all himself with his lies and his drug use. He said that, at that time, he had no faith in himself but he knew he had to do something.

At that time, Dan was not a religious or even what he would consider a spiritual man. He acknowledged, "It all began to change when I made this leap of faith to trust the process. I just embraced everything as if it were going to work. The more I did what the program said worked, the more I saw it working and started to believe in myself, in my ability to take my life back." Through tears, he said: "It was worth it. Every single day, even the hard ones, when I compare my life today to how it was when I was using, I am convinced recovery was the best thing that ever happened to me. My life was shit when I was using, lying to myself that I was in control. I wasn't in control; the drugs were. Now I am in control because I don't lie anymore and I don't have to be afraid anymore. I like myself now. I like the man I have become."

Not everyone is able to simply trust the process. It is hard to stop doing something that has been helpful to cover pain, especially when you don't know what life is going to be like without the alcohol or other drugs. If you think about what motivates you, it will help. Not wanting to face reality or the pain surrounding life's problems or the fear of stopping is surely motivation to continue to drink or use. But more important, what are the values that you want to guide you? As a man or woman, parent, friend, spouse—whatever roles you play in your life—what are the values that are important to you and how do you want to be in each of those roles? If you see yourself as religious or spiritual, what values do you want to guide you there? When you use, how do you support or go against those values? How can those values help you overcome or meet that fear that keeps you bonded to your drug use?

As the first part of embracing the process, the following exercise will help you identify the values you want to be your guide.

## Exercise 1:   Values

When you have been using drugs addictively for a long time, it is often hard to believe that you have any values that can guide you. When given the chance, however, everyone can draw on a value or two, even though it has been a long time since they honored that value. (If you cannot conjure up even one value of your own, think about someone you admire and want to be like. Use the values you think guide that person as your own for this exercise.)

List all the roles you have in life (man, woman, parent, teacher, community member, child of God, student, best friend, etc.).

_____

_____

_____

_____

_____

After each role, list the values that you want to guide you in your thoughts and actions when you are the person playing that role. Think about being in that role as if you were doing so from a healthy perspective.

## Example:

### *Role*: **Being a best friend**

(Hint: A best friend is honest, so honesty would be a guiding value.)

*Guiding Values*: be honest, be trustworthy, be emotionally available, be willing to commit time to the friendship, establish and honor boundaries, listen to my friend and share information about myself, have empathy for my friend, ask for what I need, be willing to tolerate some emotional pain for growth in the relationship—invite my friend to be honest and tell me when I am violating boundaries or going against one of my values; I can have fun without an artificial high with drugs.

Now circle the values that you have honored or that have guided you at some time in your life. With a highlighter, mark the ones that have been absent or waning when you have been using drugs.

### *Role*:

Guiding Values:

_____

_____

_____

_____

_____

_____

_____

_____

_____

### *Role*:

Guiding Values:

_____

_____

_____

_____

_____

_____

_____

_____

_____

_____

### *Role*:

Guiding Values:

_____

_____

_____

_____

_____

_____

_____

_____

_____

_____

### *Role*:

Guiding Values:

_____

_____

_____

_____

_____

_____

_____

_____

_____

How can these values help you with your process of recovery?

From your list, write down those values that you want to incorporate into your life on a daily basis. Make a copy of these on a note card to put in your purse or wallet. Make another copy to go on your bathroom mirror or to tape on the dashboard on your car—anywhere where it will be useful to see what values you want to guide your life. (If you do not want others to see this list right now, use symbols so *you* will know the meaning and can be reminded of what is important to you.) If you think it would increase your motivation to attach a goal to the values list, do that, too. For example, if you value honesty, the goal for the first week might be to be honest 75 percent of the time and to be accountable 100 percent of the time by being honest about lying each time you catch yourself telling a lie.

You might be wondering, "How can this be all that helpful? No one is without fault." You are right! No one is perfect, thank goodness. It would be very hard for the rest of us. The idea is to strive to use your values as much as possible as tools of motivation. The goal is progress, not perfection.

Sometimes it is helpful to look at the worst of the past to really understand how you have violated your values and how you want to be different. It is important in your recovery to see where there are discrepancies between how you want to be and how you in fact are when you are using drugs.

## Exercise 2:   My Ten Worst Situations

Take time now to consider the worst of your drug-using situations. List the ten worst situations you have experienced while under the influence of alcohol and/or other drugs. Some of these situations may be related to coming down from a binge or a run. Identify the value that was compromised during this situation. For each situation, record the feelings you recall having then, and the feelings you are having now as you look back at these worst or most embarrassing events.

As you make your list, don't forget to consider the following information or experiences:

- Pictures of you while using, or video and audio tapes showing you under the influence

- Blackouts, unpredictable behavior, fights with physical or emotional consequences

- Suicidal thoughts or plans

- Accident review—consider accidents you have had that were associated with drug use, or that occurred while you were under the influence

- Arrests or near arrests; breaking the law and gloating over it or feeing guilty about it

- Times you were, or could have been, caught lying, cheating, or stealing

- Loss of driver's license or professional license

- Getting expelled or kicked out of school or a training program

- Increased arguing or fighting with loved ones or co-workers

- In debt, in or near bankruptcy

- Unsuccessful attempts to stop or cut down

- Putting yourself in high-risk situations to satisfy your addiction

- Lost jobs, opportunities

- A loved one's description of you when you were using and they weren't

1. Situation:_____

   _____

   Values compromised:_____
   Feelings then:_____
   Feelings now:_____

2. Situation:_____

   _____

   Values compromised:_____
   Feelings then:_____
   Feelings now:_____

3. Situation:_____

   _____

   Values compromised:_____
   Feelings then:_____
   Feelings now:_____

4. Situation:_____

   _____

   Values compromised:_____
   Feelings then:_____
   Feelings now:_____

5. Situation:_____

_____

   Values compromised:_____

   Feelings then:_____

   Feelings now:_____

6. Situation:_____

_____

   Values compromised:_____

   Feelings then:_____

   Feelings now:_____

7. Situation:_____

_____

   Values compromised:_____

   Feelings then:_____

   Feelings now:_____

8. Situation:_____

_____

   Values compromised:_____

   Feelings then:_____

   Feelings now:_____

9. Situation:_____

_____

   Values compromised:_____

   Feelings then:_____

   Feelings now:_____

10.   Situation:_____

_____

Values compromised:_____
Feelings then:_____
Feelings now:_____

After you have finished, you may wish to rank these situations. This will help you to focus on where and when you have experienced the greatest powerlessness and unmanageability. If you prepare a Step One (of the Twelve Steps of AA and similar programs) this list will be useful.

Some people think the twelve-step program for drug addiction is a cop out because recovering people state they are powerless over alcohol (or other drugs and behaviors). Not true*! Being powerless does not mean you have no responsibility.* It means that in the past your efforts to stop or cut down were fruitless. *You are not powerless over your behavior.* Becoming aware of how the addictive behavior has had power over your life is one of the important steps to recovery. Knowing the skills for dealing with cravings and how to stop using, as well as having the motivation to change your behavior, are significant in the process of recovery.

## Exercise 3:   Powerlessness Inventory

In this exercise, list as many examples as possible that show how you have been powerless to stop your substance abuse. Being "powerless" is believing you cannot stop a certain behavior, despite obvious consequences. Think about all the attempts you have made to stop or to control your use. How did you bargain with yourself about starting to use again? You may want to refer back to Chapter One, Exercise 3, to see the Twenty Excuses to Use Exercise for hints about this bargaining behavior. Identify at least twenty-five examples of being powerless over the disease. Unearthing as many examples as you can directly improves the degree of insight you develop into your substance use.

You do not have to complete this task in one sitting. Add examples over time, perhaps using a different color of ink each time you return to the task. By finding as many examples as possible, you will have added significantly to the depth of your understanding of your own powerlessness and your ability to overcome this predicament by creating new ways to solve problems you believed you could do nothing about. Understanding powerlessness is essential to overcoming your denial of the seriousness of your substance problem.

When you finish this inventory, discuss it with your group or therapist.

*Example*: Karen said she would leave me if I used narcotic pain pills without her knowledge and a doctor's prescription. I used some anyway and lied repeatedly to her when I knew she knew the truth.

1. _____

_____

_____


2. _____

_____

_____


3. _____

_____

_____


4. _____

_____

_____


5. _____

_____

_____

6. _____

_____

_____

7. _____

_____

_____

8. _____

_____

_____

9. _____

_____

_____

10. _____

_____

_____

## Exercise 4:   Unmanageability Inventory

In this exercise, list as many examples as possible of how your drug use has been unmanageable from time to time. "Unmanageability" means the ways your substance use created chaos, problems, or harm to you or someone else. Many addicts are able to control their drug use some of the time, but most addicts can't _reliably_ manage their addiction. They cannot usually predict when using would make life unmanageable. Try to identify at least twenty-five examples.

You do not have to complete this task in one sitting. By giving as many examples as possible, you will have added significantly to the depth of your understanding of your own unmanageability and your ability to overcome this dilemma. Understanding the instances of unmanageability is essential for discovering ways to build healthier solutions in your life.

*Example*: One Saturday night I went to "the Castle," our local hangout, with John and Bill to dance and drink. I don't know how many shots of tequila I had had when someone offered me ecstasy. I don't remember what happened after that. When I awoke the next morning, I was in bed with a woman whose name I didn't know. I had no idea where I was. When she woke up she told me *I'd asked* to spend the night with her.

1. _____

_____

2. _____

_____

3. _____

_____

4. _____

_____

5. _____

_____

6. _____

   _____

7. _____

   _____

8. _____

   _____

9. _____

   _____

10. _____

    _____

11. _____

    _____

12. _____

    _____

13. _____

_____

14. _____

_____

15. _____

_____

16. _____

_____

17. _____

_____

18. _____

_____

19. _____

_____

20. _____

_____

21. _____

   _____

22. _____

   _____

23. _____

   _____

24. _____

   _____

25. _____

   _____

When you finish this inventory, discuss it with your group or therapist. Be sure to discuss what you had to do to cover up these episodes.

# Impact on Relationships

How would you feel if your spouse or life partner were involved in an affair with another person? Imagine that your partner seems distracted when you try to have a conversation and that he or she has unexplained mood swings—but you don't know why. Imagine that your partner spends a lot of time involved in other activities away from home, that your bank account has withdrawals that your partner can't really account for, that your partner forgets promises he or she made to you, and he or she no longer seems interested in your children. Even if you don't know the details, it's clear that your partner's attention is focused elsewhere.

This could be a description of a person engaged in an extramarital affair—and it is! But rather than another person, the "lover" might be the bottle, the needle, or the spoon. The bottom line is that an addict's primary relationship is no longer with the partner but rather with their drug of choice. One way of distinguishing an enjoyable, life-enhancing activity from an addiction is to determine what it does to the rest of your life. Does it expand your life and allow you to engage in new activities, to make new friends, and to increase your enthusiasm with your primary relationship? Or does your involvement with it cause you to pull away from your family, give up your old friends, forget about exercising and eating right, and neglect your career. When your addiction becomes your highest priority, your relationship with your partner and your family is sure to suffer.

## Exercise 5:   Impact of Drug Use on My Relationships

Take a few moments to think about how your relationships have been affected by your drinking and drugging. Make a list of specific incidents. Next to each one, write down how the other person reacted and how you believe he or she felt about your behavior. Finally, write down how you now feel about that incident. For example,

> On my birthday three months ago, my husband suggested that we eat at home, that we would make a special occasion of it, and that he would take care of everything. All I had to do was come from work by 6 P.M.. That day, my boss chewed me out for something, getting me very upset. On the way home, I stopped for a drink with a girlfriend. We polished off a couple of bottles of wine, and next thing I knew it was 9 o'clock. I rushed home, almost getting a speeding ticket. When I got there, my husband was no-where to be seen, and his car was gone. On the table was a gourmet dinner he'd ordered from the best restaurant in town, now cold and soggy; candles that had burned to the bottom and then gone out; and a note from my husband saying that the kids were at my mom's for the night.

> When my husband returned from the long drive he'd taken to cool off, he was still really steamed. I apologized and told him that I'd had to stay late at work. He yelled at

me that he was tired of my "forgetting" important en-
gagements and that he was through doing nice things for
me. He spent the night on the sofa in the living room.

I'm sure he felt rejected and unimportant, and that I just
didn't care about him.

Now I realize that he was right—my actions showed him
that indeed he was not as important to me as my drinking. I also showed him I was a liar. I feel ashamed about
my behavior. We had many such episodes; it's amazing he
stayed around as long as he did.

How my drug use has affected my relationships with others (spouse or
partner, children, other relatives, friends, colleagues) :

1. _____

   _____

   _____

   _____

   _____

   _____

2. _____

   _____

   _____

   _____

   _____

   _____

3. _____

_____

_____

_____

_____

_____

4. _____

_____

_____

_____

_____

_____

5. _____

_____

_____

_____

_____

_____

6. _____

_____

_____

_____

_____

_____

7. _____

_____

_____

_____

_____

_____

8. _____

_____

_____

_____

_____

_____

9. _____

_____

_____

_____

_____

_____

10. _____

_____

_____

_____

_____

# Impact on One's Career

In June 2002, two veteran America West Airlines pilots reacted with anger when they were told at the Miami Airport security area that they could not carry their full coffee cups onto the plane they were about to board and fly to Phoenix, Arizona. A security guard smelled alcohol on their breaths. Breathalyzer tests confirmed that they both had significantly elevated blood alcohol levels, above the 0.08 legal limit in Florida. In a highly publicized report, both pilots were immediately arrested, fired by the airline, and had their pilots' licenses revoked by the Federal Aviation Administration. Two long, previously unblemished careers were instantly down the drain.

Remember the *Exxon Valdez* oil spill in Prince William Sound in Alaska? In 1989, a huge oil tanker ran aground and spilled more than 11 million gallons of crude oil into one of the largest and most important estuaries in North America. Ninety-nine miles of shoreline in Prince William Sound were heavily covered in oil, and an additional 285 miles were at least lightly covered in oil. About 250,000 birds and thousands of other animals were killed. It took four years and $2.1 billion to clean up most of the mess, but as of 2001 many miles of contaminated shoreline still existed. The captain of the ship, who had a long record of alcohol abuse, was charged with piloting a vessel under the influence of alcohol. He was eventually acquitted by an Alaskan jury, but there was much speculation that alcohol was involved.

Professionals who risk their jobs because of their drug use tend to be in the advanced stages of their addictive disorder. Long before that, they usually have experienced negative consequences in their personal lives. Most often, the job is the last part of their life to be affected. Taking these risks represents a significant lapse in judgment.

## Exercise 6:   How Drug Use Affected My Job

Think about any situations where your drug use affected your job. It doesn't have to be in a dramatic way, such as causing a plane crash, an oil spill, or a botched surgery. Ask yourself: Have I taken time off from work, or been late to work, because of my drug use? Have I done a poor job because I was either under the influence of a chemical or recovering from the effects of too much use the night before? How much of my work time have I spent obsessing about the next time I could use or trying to obtain my drugs? Have I made a poor decision that had a negative impact on other employees or on the company's profits? Have I behaved inappropriately at work (such as making off-color or demeaning jokes or comments or displaying excessive anger) because I was under the influence? Have I taken risks with other people's lives while under the influence or because I was distracted?

Make a list of any such circumstances you can recall. Next to your item, write down what was the consequence, if any. Include consequences for you (including excessive worry and guilt), consequences for others on the job, and the impact on your company's performance.

_____

_____

_____

_____

_____

_____

_____

_____

_____

_____

_____

_____

_____

_____

_____

# Impact on One's Soul

Rose was sexually abused by her father from the time she was 11 until she ran away from home at the age of 16. By 22, she was married and had two small children. She was also a full-blown alcoholic and smoked two packs of cigarettes per day. This was her way of coping with her past. By 25, she was divorced and a single parent. For the next eight years, her primary relationship was with alcohol and cigarettes. On many occasions she left her children alone in the house while she went to a bar or else brought home bottles of whiskey and drank until she passed out. At age 33, after a fire set by the cigarette she was holding when she passed out nearly killed her and her children, she found Alcoholics Anonymous (AA) and sobered up. Later, she became an alcoholism counselor—a very good one. However, she was never able to forgive herself for the parenting her children had lacked during her drinking years and the risk she placed them in by exposing them to the hazards of second-hand smoke (and the fire). She made amends to them on numerous occasions, and they repeatedly expressed their for-giveness, but deep inside she continued to believe she was a worthless person and a horrible parent. She blamed herself for every misstep her children took. She also continued to blame herself for having agreed to have intercourse with her father during her teen years. Despite being told that sexual abuse of a child is never the child's fault, she kept telling herself she was old enough to have known better and to have been able to resist him. Her soul had been deeply damaged.

It is easier for most people to recognize the damage they have inflicted on others than to realize that they have hurt themselves as well. Most people, except those who have no conscience, feel good about themselves when they behave with integrity and do good, and feel bad when they don't measure up to their own internal standards. All too often addicts do *not* measure up, with the result that they beat themselves up, repeatedly reminding themselves of how worthless they are and how undeserving of love and affection from others. If you were the victim of abuse, someone else started the damage to your soul. If you have continued the abuse by using drugs or behaving in a way that harms you and those you care about, you have continued to damage your soul.

All of the exercises in this book have been designed to raise your awareness of the impact of addiction on your life. We frequently ask people what will happen if they continue to use drugs in a year, five years, ten years, and so on. Without fail, those problem drug users speculate that they will be dead, in jail or that they will have lost everything if they continue to use. Depending on whether fear or strength motivates you, complete one of the following exercises. If you don't know yet what motivates you, do both and see which one has the most power right now in your life.

## Exercise 7A:   Obituary

In this exercise, you will have continued to use alcohol and/or other drugs. Based on what you have learned so far, let's say that your drug use progressed and perhaps you also engaged in other addictive behaviors that contributed to greater pain for you and your family. This results in a car accident in which you are killed. Let's say this happens within the next ten years. How old would you be at your death? How old would your children be?

What hopes have you not had an opportunity to fulfill?

_____

_____

What activities have you not been able to accomplish?

_____

_____

Who is left behind? Who would grieve for you? Who would attend your funeral?

_____

_____

Now think about who would speak at your funeral and what they would say about you. Write out what you would hear them thinking about you as they prepared this eulogy and then write what they would say at your funeral. Feel free to use your journal if you need more space.

_____

_____

_____

_____

_____

_____

_____

_____

_____

_____

_____

_____

_____

_____

_____

_____

_____

_____

_____

_____

_____

_____

_____

_____

What was it like to see and hear what this would be like? How can this image assist you in your recovery process?

## Exercise 7B:   85th Birthday

In this exercise, imagine that your efforts to honor yourself and your values have resulted in learning recovery skills and staying motivated. Your efforts have worked. It is now your 85th birthday, and you have had many years of an addiction-free life. Your family has planned a special birthday celebration.

Who is present?

_____

_____

What are you grateful about and for?

_____

_____

What has motivated you that you have shared with those people who are special in your life?

_____

_____

Who will speak at your birthday celebration?

_____

_____

What will they be thinking about you when they write the speech celebrating your birthday?

_____

_____

Write out the speech you would hope to hear at this celebration.

_____

_____

_____

_____

_____

_____

_____

_____

_____

_____

_____

_____

_____

_____

_____

_____

_____

_____

_____

_____

_____

What was it like to see yourself at your 85th birthday celebration?

_____

_____

_____

_____

What about this event can contribute to your recovery process?

_____

_____

_____

_____

Now review the two exercises and reflect on how each exercise can motivate you.

# First-Order and Second-Order Change

As you can see, the focus has been on your values as well as on the ways your addiction has cost you. This is easier with the help of a spiritual connection or higher power of some sort, therapist, twelve-step meetings, a sponsor, supportive family members who are working on their own changes, and someone helping to monitor your efforts. Nonetheless, being able to make change is primarily related to how you want life to be different and what you want to do about it. How you think about changing is an important part of how motivated you will remain during the tougher parts of the recovery process. If you change only because you don't want to lose your job, or spouse, or kids, you will soon find that you are stuck in what we call first-order change. After some time, you will start to get mad about the demands that others are making on you, and resentment will begin to grow. Sure enough, when resentment is taking up space in your head, the addict voice that doesn't want you to change will find some way to contaminate your thinking process. On the other hand, if you are changing because you like being the kind of person whose behavior reflects healthy values, it is much

| **First-Order of Change** *Addicts Believe:* | **Second-Order of Change** *Recovering People Believe:* |
|---|---|
| No one will know what I am doing. | I will know that I am going against my values. |
| I don't need anyone, I can handle this myself. | I want other people in my life. By being honest, I invite others to trust me. |
| I always figure out a solution. | Sometimes there are things I cannot control. |
| No one understands me. | If I am honest, I invite others to understand me. |
| What she doesn't know won't hurt her. | Addict behavior hurts me and the people I care about. |
| Things are not so bad. I can stop anytime I want. | If I continue to use, things will continue to get worse. |

more likely that your motivation will remain high and that you will be making changes because of genuine belief. With some skill building and practice, you can manage your emotions and your behavior.

# Skills Needed for Each Kind of Change

### Exercise 8:   Cost-Benefit Analysis

Based on your work thus far in this book, complete the decision-making matrix below. In the upper-right-hand quadrant, list the positive reasons for continuing to use drugs. In the upper-left-hand quadrant, list the negative reasons for continuing to use. In the lower-right-hand quadrant, list the positive reasons for stopping your drug use. In the lower-left-hand quadrant, list the negative reasons for stopping your drug use.

## Decision-Making Matrix

| **Negative Reasons to Use Drugs** | **Positive Reasons to Use Drugs** |
|---|---|
| | |
| **Negative Reasons to Stop Using Drugs** | **Positive Reasons to Stop Using Drugs** |
| | |

How can this help you in your recovery process? Are there other ways to get your needs met—the role that drugs played in the past? What skills do you need to learn in order to get those needs met?

_____

_____

_____

_____

_____

_____

# Process of Recovery over Time

We may have made this process sound easy. Life is as easy as you make it. That goes for recovery, too. If you embrace it and take it *one day at a time,* you can get through this. The journey is hard, however, and it can be helpful to know a little of what to expect during the first stages of recovery.

There have been few longitudinal studies on the process of recovery over time. In his book *The Natural History of Alcohol Revisited,* George Vaillant observes that, as expected, better physical health is one of the consequences of alcohol abstinence. Probably the best study was *Don't Call It Love,* by Patrick Carnes, 1991 on sex addicts, 42 percent of whom had concurrent chemical dependency. His observations on these addicts can undoubtedly be extrapolated to those who are solely chemically dependent. Carnes found that during the first year of recovery, most slips, if they occurred at all, took place in the second six months. This was also the worst period for health of the entire first five years of recovery: Accidents, illnesses, and visits to physicians occurred most frequently during the second six months of recovery (Carnes, p. 186).

During the second and third years, things got better in many areas: There were improvements in financial and career status and in one's ability to cope with stress, friendships, self-image, and spirituality. The following two years were a time of repairing significant relationships—those with one's spouse or partner, children, parents, and siblings. Life satisfaction generally improved significantly during the fourth and fifth years.

In other words, the first year is not easy for addicts. One of the most common emotions is grief—grief over the loss of one's "friend," the drug, and grief over the damage and pain caused to oneself and one's family and friends. You may need to make amends and reparations for the adverse consequences of your drinking and using. During this year, you need to establish a new life pattern, negotiate with your spouse or partner (if you have one) about your meeting attendance, and practice honesty. None of these are easy, but, if you persist, you will be rewarded.

As we stated in the Preface, we have added information at the end of the book about the 12 Step program of Alcoholics Anonymous (and about other twelve-step groups for all behavioral and drug addictions). At the end of the book is a list of tasks that are useful in helping individuals stay on task through the first few years of recovery. Of course it is important to remember, in highly stressful times, that you care more for yourself, not less, no matter how long you have been in recovery.

In the next two chapters, we will discuss the damage from your behavior. As you complete the exercises there, it will be helpful to have the list of the guiding values you have created in this chapter to help you make decisions about how you want to be accountable for your behavior. Being accountable is painful AND healing.

## Step One

In the 12 Steps of Alcohol Anonymous, Step One says:

> *We admitted that our lives were powerless over alcohol—that our lives had become unmanageable.*

The information you collected in this chapter is what you will need to complete Step One in a traditional twelve step program. Review this information with your sponsor, and make a plan to present this information to members of your support group.

## References

Carnes, Patrick. *Don't Call it Love* (New York: Bantam, 1991), p.35.

Vaillant, George. *The Natural History of Alcohol Revisited* (Cambridge, Mass: Harvard University Press, 1995), p. 276.

# CHAPTER FIVE: Damage to the Body from Drug Abuse

**damage** n. *injury or harm to a person or thing resulting in a loss of strength or integrity*

An early step to addiction recovery is to recognize the damage your behaviors have caused you. By completing the exercises in the earlier chapters, you have already begun to think about the consequences of your addiction to your body, psyche, relationships, career, and soul, as well as to other people. In this chapter, we will explore in greater depth the short- and long-term physical effects of your substance(s) of choice.

# Damage to the Body and Mind

Progressive use of any mood-altering substance imposes harm on your body and mind. Rarely is this harm appreciated early in the course of your attachment to the drug; if it did, you would have been strongly motivated to stop in order to avoid direct harm. However, most forms of harm that are borne by the body and mind occur subtly over long periods of time. The linkage of cause and effect is far more difficult for you to discern. In addition, the body and mind are created with a significant amount of "excess capacity" to perform their functions. For example, one kidney is enough to adequately cleanse the body of waste products. One quarter of the liver is enough to metabolize chemicals, and the liver can quickly regenerate itself. This is why people can donate a kidney or part of a liver to others, yet remain healthy. Much of the harm from substance use is hidden as the progression of addiction eats away at this excess capacity.

The great tragedy in drug addiction is precisely this: By the time drug use has moved through experimentation, social use, and controlled use, to the point where the unmanageability and consequences of use can no longer be denied, the harm done to the body and mind has progressed as well. This harm moves from stress upon the body/mind, through reversible effects, and on to specific patterns of damage in multiple organs. Following are descriptions of the short- and long-term medical consequences of abuse of several commonly used drugs. This list is not meant to be exhaustive or complete.

# Alcohol

<u>Short-term effects</u>: On many college campuses, fraternity-hazing rites include consuming a great deal of alcohol. On multiple occasions, young people have died after drinking far more than their body was used to handling. This was a result of alcohol's sedative effects. But alcohol is also a disinhibitor, impairing the drinker's ability to make good decisions. The person might get into an argument that results in a physical fight, or he might drive a car unsafely and thereby injure himself or others. A large proportion of emergency room visits are related to alcohol consumption. In chronic high-level alcohol consumers, blood clotting is sometimes impaired; if they get into an accident, they will bleed more heavily. If they have head trauma, they are more likely than nondrinkers to sustain a subdural hematoma, which is bleeding into the brain, a potentially fatal event.

Alcohol is one of the few drugs whose withdrawal syndrome can be fatal. Most chronic drinkers who stop experience only tremor, anxiety, elevated heart rate, and insomnia, but some develop fever, seizures, and hallucinations, and some of them die.

<u>Long-term effects</u>: Long-term alcoholics are usually nutritionally deficient because they get most of their calories from alcohol. Other medical problems in long-term drinkers occur in the following organ systems:

- Brain and nervous system:

    "Blackouts"—periods of time the person does not remember although he may have appeared to function normally.

Wernicke-Korsakoff syndrome—a type of dementia caused by alcohol. The person has memory loss, which he attempts to cover by making up stories.

Peripheral neuropathy—numbness and painful burning in the feet and hands.

- Gastrointestinal (GI) tract:

    Gastritis—inflammation and pain of the stomach lining.

    Gastrointestinal bleeding—can be caused by gastritis or by the bursting of enlarged veins in the esophagus. High pressures in other parts of the GI tract, caused by alcohol damage, cause the veins to become enlarged.

    Acute and chronic pancreatitis (inflammation of the pancreas)—patients have recurrent severe abdominal pain, nausea, and vomiting, which may require hospitalization.

    Alcoholic hepatitis—a severe inflammation of the liver. With time, the inflammation becomes *cirrhosis*, an irreversible breakdown of liver tissue, which is replaced by nonfunctional fibrous tissue. Although the liver has a lot of "excess capacity," eventually this capacity is exceeded, and only a liver transplant will save the person. The ethics of giving liver transplants to alcoholics is controversial, but there is general consensus that, to qualify for a transplant, the person must have stopped drinking.

- The vascular system:

    Hypertension—elevated blood pressure is a common effect of recurrent alcohol consumption.

    Enlarged red blood cells—these indicate some damage to the bone marrow, where blood cells are formed.

- The endocrine system and metabolism:

    Alcohol use decreases the production of both male and female sex hormones. Women develop menstrual irregularities or stop having periods altogether; men's sperm count can become lower, and they may experience erectile dysfunction.

Uric acid levels are often elevated, leading to episodes of gout, a painful inflammation of the great toes and other areas.

- Cancer:

   Alcohol abuse increases the risks of several types of cancer—including pancreas, liver, stomach, esophagus, colon, and mouth cancers.

- Pregnancy:

   Women who continue drinking heavily during their pregnancy are at risk of giving birth to babies with fetal alcohol syndrome (FAS). This syndrome, present in up to 12,000 babies born each year, is a combination of distinct facial abnormalities, growth deficiency, and evidence of brain abnormalities. The child may have poor motor skills and hand-eye coordination, and she may also have a complex pattern of behavioral and learning problems, including difficulties with memory, attention, and judgment. FAS is considered the most common nonhereditary cause of mental retardation. It is permanent. And it is completely preventable.

# Opioids (Narcotics)

Opiates are drugs derived from opium, such as morphine and codeine, and semisynthetic compounds created from them, such as heroin. The term *opioid* is broader than *opiate*, including fully synthetic drugs such as methadone, as well as all drugs that bind to the opiate receptors in the body, whether they activate or inhibit the pleasure centers, and whether they are taken into the body or produced by the body.

Opioids are the most potent drug class available for pain relief. When prescribed by a doctor for this purpose and used as directed, they are very effective and remarkably safe. They do not damage any organ. Their main side effects are nausea and vomiting, sedation, and constipation. Patients generally develop a tolerance to the sedative and nauseating effects of opioids (meaning that these side effects go away), but the tendency to constipation continues as long as the drugs are taken. When people take prescribed opioids for pain, they generally do *not* develop a tolerance to the pain-relieving effects of these drugs. This means that, once they have reached an adequate pain-relieving dose of the prescribed opioid, they are likely to be able to stay on the same dose for a long time. If they eventually need more, it's probably because their disease has gotten worse.

Thousands of people in the United States take methadone daily for many years as part of their recovery from narcotic addiction. These people are healthy and can lead normal lives. Their supervised methadone use does not cause their body any damage. Babies born to methadone-using women do not experience any damage, except that they may be born addicted and need to be weaned off it.

It's a different story when opioids are abused.

When heroin and other narcotics are obtained on the street, the quantity that is put into the body is often uncertain. The most serious immediate side effect is respiratory depression if the user has inadvertently used a larger amount than he realized. This is the usual cause of death from narcotic use. If your drug of choice is one of the prescription combination drugs that contain Tylenol (acetaminophen), such as Percocet, Lorcet, or Vicodin, the biggest risk is liver damage from the acetaminophen. People have died of liver failure from taking too many pills containing Tylenol. If, however, you take drugs, such as Percodan, that are a combination of oxycodone and aspirin, you can get seriously ill from an overdose of the aspirin component. Certain opioids, including Demerol (meperidine), Darvon (propoxyphene), and Talwin (pentazocine), are metabolized in the body to form compounds that can produce seizures. Large doses of any of these drugs can result in seizures.

When narcotics are injected, the injection process itself can produce serious medical problems. The most serious is the transmission of the HIV and hepatitis viruses when dirty needles are used. Additionally, subcutaneous injection ("skin-popping") done without first disinfecting the skin can result in abscesses. Depending on where the drug is injected, abscesses can be so serious as to require hospitalization for intravenous antibiotic treatment and sometimes even surgery.

Withdrawal from narcotic abuse has a well-recognized syndrome, which includes abdominal cramps and other pains, diarrhea, vomiting, excessive tearing, and goose bumps. These symptoms are very uncomfortable but are not dangerous.

Apart from the continued risk of all these acute medical problems, there are no specific ill effects on the body when narcotic addiction continues for years. The worst effects are on the addict's relationships, career, finances, risk of arrest, and risk of being injured or killed because of the person's lifestyle. Not surprisingly, when addicts take a moment to reflect on their life, they may become depressed.

## Cocaine and Amphetamines

Because cocaine is a local anesthetic (a numbing agent, like lidocaine [Xylocaine]) and a vasoconstrictor (it narrows blood vessels), it is used by physicians to examine the inside of the nose.

Short-term effects: Even when used nonmedically in "usual" doses, cocaine can be fatal because it can cause abnormal heart rhythms (arrhythmias) that result in sudden death. This is apparently what happened to University of Maryland basketball player, Len Bias, who was found dead at the age of 22 in 1986, with cocaine in his body. Cocaine users can experience high blood pressure, chest pain, heart attacks, and strokes. These effects might be caused by cocaine's ability to constrict blood vessels, thereby depriving organs of needed blood. People on cocaine binges may stay awake for days and develop paranoia and even psychosis. When cocaine is injected or smoked, seizures can develop.

Cocaine does not have a well-defined withdrawal syndrome but, like most drugs, when someone whose body is habituated to using it stops, the effects on the body are the opposite of those seen during drug use. Because cocaine and amphetamines are stimulants, stopping use after a binge is followed by a "crash." The person feels fatigued, exhausted, and depressed, and he believes the solution is to use more.

Long-term effects: When the user repeatedly inhales cocaine through the nose (snorts), constriction of the blood vessels in the nose can lead to destruction of the membrane (septum) between the nostrils and a resultant hole there. This is an easy way to diagnose some chronic cocaine addicts. The same mechanism can result in inadequate blood supply to the gas-trointestinal tract, which can severely damage the intestines and the liver. There is some controversy over whether cocaine is harmful to the babies of addicted pregnant women. Part of the difficulty is that these women tend to use a combination of addictive drugs.

The mood-altering effects of amphetamines resemble those of cocaine, but they are much longer lasting. Their toxicity is similar, too.

# Marijuana

The source of marijuana is the *Cannabis sativa* plant, which contains many psychoactive chemicals known as cannabinoids. The most potent one is THC, or delta-9-tetrahydrocannabinol, the greatest concentration of which is found in the flowering tops of the plants. There is now some research in animals showing that THC is a weak pain reliever that can improve the efficacy of opioids when both are used together. A product called Marinol contains synthetic THC in tablet form. This medication can be prescribed by doctors to control nausea and vomiting caused by chemo-therapeutic agents used in treating cancer and as an appetite stimulant in AIDS patients. It is also used to treat people with glaucoma, an eye disease.

Marijuana and hashish are generally smoked as *joints* (loosely rolled cigarettes), or as *blunts* (packed into hollowed-out commercial cigars). The peak effect is felt within ten to thirty minutes, and effects may last for two or three hours. These often depend upon the expectation of the person using the drug. Low doses tend to induce a feeling of well-being and relaxation. This state of intoxication may not be noticeable to an observer. However, driving, occupational, and household accidents can result from a distortion of time and space and impaired coordination that is present even after the effects of the marijuana seem to have worn off. When used repeat-edly, marijuana can cause an "amotivational syndrome." The user is no longer interested in putting effort into education, career, or relationships. His main interest is in sitting around and smoking.

Stronger doses intensify reactions, and users may experience shifting sensory imagery, rapid mood swings, fragmentary thoughts with altered sense of self-identity, impaired memory, and a dulling attention despite an *illusion* of heightened insight. High doses may result in image distortion, loss of personal identity, and fantasies and hallucinations.

Another problem with marijuana is that, because its sale is illegal, you can never be sure of exactly what you will be putting into your body. Marijuana is sometimes laced with PCP (phencyclidine, "angel dust") to make its effects more potent. PCP is a powerful hallucinogen that commonly causes psychotic reactions. The unexpected effects of PCP can frighten and panic the user. You might feel superhuman strength and invulnerability, and therefore you might take risks that could result in harm to yourself. One PCP-using young man once climbed out his third-story window and began to swing on the adjacent power line. He apparently thought he was Tarzan. Unfortunately, he lost his grip and fell to his death. In the past, some marijuana was contaminated with paraquat, an herbicide used to kill weeds while growing the Cannabis plants. The paraquat produced severe lung toxicity when the marijuana was smoked.

The ease with which people can obtain marijuana makes it a desirable first drug, along with nicotine, for young people, and it is often thought to be a "gateway" drug to more dangerous drugs. Most long-term narcotic users began their drug careers by using nicotine and marijuana.

Marijuana metabolites are stored in the fat cells in the body for long periods of time, making detection of the drug very easy through drug screens. The risk to the lungs of long-term users is similar to that of nicotine users—trouble breathing due to bronchitis, emphysema, and bronchial asthma.

# Polydrug Abuse

Although many people abuse or are addicted only to alcohol, it is increasingly common for users to combine mood-altering drugs. In some cases, the effects of the drugs are similar, and the goal is to increase the same effect. This is why alcohol may be combined with benzodiazepines (such as Valium or Librium). When several brain depressants are used together, there is an increased risk of sedation and respiratory depression. In other cases, one drug is used to combat the effect of the other. For example, cocaine (an upper) is combined with alcohol (a downer). When these two drugs are combined, however, a third psychoactive drug, cocaethylene, is formed in the body, which can produce increased toxicity. When cocaine and heroin are combined (a "speedball"), the risk of seizure is increased. Other combinations seem to be taken randomly, as in when someone is offered various drugs at a party and accepts whatever is offered.

# Tobacco

It is ironic that the most dangerous and most commonly abused substances in the world—tobacco and alcohol—are both legal in the United States. The risks of tobacco smoking are so well known that we will mention them only briefly here. Cigarettes contain many carcinogens (cancer-causing chemicals). In the United States, 30 percent of *all* cancer deaths are attributed to tobacco use. Tobacco is by far the major cause of lung cancer worldwide. Smoking cigarettes and chewing tobacco both increase the risk of cancers of the larynx and mouth. Pipe and cigar smokers are at high risk for cancers of the lining of the mouth, and pipe smokers are also at increased risk of lip cancer. Long-term exposure to second-hand smoke in the environment has increased the risk of lung cancer in nonsmokers by 30 percent and accounts for about 3,000 cases of lung cancer in the United States each year.

Cigarette smoking is the most consistent risk factor for cancer of the pancreas. It is also associated with increased risk of cervical cancer. Tobacco use accounts for one-third to one-half of all bladder cancers diagnosed in the United States. In addition to increasing the risk of many cancers, smoking greatly increases the likelihood of heart attacks, strokes, and peripheral vascular disease (blockages in major arteries in the legs).

Have you ever noticed that heavy smokers often look older than their age? That's because smoking ages the skin and accelerates the formation of wrinkles.

With all these terrible effects, why would anyone continue smoking? The answer, unfortunately, is that smoking is one of the hardest addictions to quit. Many people who have successfully overcome an alcohol addiction say that quitting smoking is much harder than quitting drinking. There is a high correlation between smoking and using other drugs. For example, a much higher percentage of drinkers than nondrinkers smoke. Alcoholics and drug addicts who continue to smoke have a harder time remaining abstinent from their drug addiction because smoking stimulates their brains to continue craving the other drugs.

## Exercise 1:  Medical Problems from Drug Use

Have you suffered any medical problems as a result of your drug use? Make a list of these effects. Don't forget psychiatric or emotional consequences! And don't forget physical injuries. For each problem, write down whether this was short term or long term, how it was treated, and what is its status today.

_____

_____

_____

_____

_____

_____

_____

_____

_____

_____

_____

_____

In the next chapter, we will turn to the types of damage done by drug abuse to relationships, career, and the soul, and we will begin to examine how to control the damage.

## References

Brick, John and Erickson, Carlton K. *Drugs, the Brain, and Behavior.* (New York: Hawthorn Medical Press, 1998)

Li, Frederick P. and Peters, Edward S. Cancer epidemiology and prevention. In Dale, David C. & Federman, Daniel D. (eds.) Scientific American Medicine, Section 12, Chapter 1. 1998. New York: Scientific American Inc.

Wartenberg, Alan A. Medical syndromes associated with specific drugs. In Miller, N.S. (ed), Principles of Addiction Medicine (Chevy Chase, Md: American Society of Addiction Medicine, 1994), Section 5, Chapter 2.

# CHAPTER SIX: Recognizing and Limiting Damage to Relationships, Career, and the Soul

**limit** v. *to confine within bounds*

After completing the exercise in Chapter 5, you might think that the worst damage from drug abuse and dependency is that which the body sustains. However, when addicts finally recognize that their lives have become unmanageable, the reasons are much more likely to be related to effects of the addiction on their relationships, career, and their own soul.

> Nelson, 32, was an up-and-coming stockbroker. In college, he had partied on weekends, drinking excessively and using marijuana and cocaine recreationally, but after getting a good job and marrying his long-time girlfriend, Nancy, he had settled down. Nancy was an administrator for a health-maintenance plan. Nelson worked hard and successfully during the week, and on weekends both of them enjoyed their comfortable suburban house and social activities. Nelson's drinking and drugging days seemed to be a thing of the long-ago past.

> Nancy and Nelson were expecting their first baby when the stock market began a downward slide. Having recommended technology stocks to his clients, he was besieged with worried, angry, and upset clients whose portfolios were losing up to half of their value. The experts were advising people to ride out the current

situation. Nelson and his associates were increasingly stressed out as they helplessly watched the value of their clients' accounts continue to drop.

One day George, an associate of Nelson's, invited him for a drink after work. When George produced a packet of cocaine and invited Nelson to share it, Nelson inhaled a line without even thinking, and for the first time in months his worries seemed to melt. He felt so good that he contacted George's dealer to obtain his own supply. Pretty soon he could hardly wait for the end of another stressful day at the office, so that he could get into the car, find a quiet place to park, and escape into a cocaine-induced euphoria. He'd usually get home very late, but he explained to Nancy that it was because he had to work longer hours.

After a few weeks it no longer seemed to matter so much what was happening to his clients' accounts. He was reprimanded twice for sloppy performance, but he just couldn't seem to focus on his job. Dissatisfied with Nelson, some of his clients switched to other brokers at his firm. Meanwhile, Nancy was becoming increasingly upset that, as her due date approached, Nelson seemed less and less interested in their relationship. One day Nelson's supervisor told him he was fired—his work performance was unacceptable, and he had ignored earlier warnings.

When Nelson arrived home late that evening after snorting more than the usual amount of cocaine, Nancy confronted him with the latest bank statement, asking for an explanation for some recent large withdrawals from their joint account. Nelson became angry, and replied, "You're not my mother! I can spend my money any way I want!"

Nancy burst into tears. "I just can't take any more of this!" she cried. "You haven't been there for me ever since I got pregnant. It's as though you don't want the baby—or me!" She ran upstairs, threw some clothes into a suitcase, and drove away.

The next morning, Nancy called Nelson at the office, intending to tell him that she was staying at her mother's house. She was shocked to hear from the receptionist that Nelson was no longer working there. When she reached him at their home, she told him it was clear he was in the midst of a crisis and that she'd decided to stay with her mother at least until after the baby's birth; after that, she would consider returning only if Nelson would get some help for his problem, whatever is was. Nelson realized that his cocaine addiction had already cost him his job and was about to cost him his marriage as well. He realized he had also lost his self-esteem and his own soul. It was time to make some changes.

Nelson started out as a self-confident young man who thought he could handle all his problems by himself. Instead of sharing them with his friends and wife and asking for help and support, he sought a solution in drugs. The solution only ended up multiplying his problems. By lying and keeping secrets from Nancy, he damaged their relationship, perhaps permanently.

You may have damaged your marriage or primary relationship by lying and keeping secrets, by having sex with people outside your marriage, by being unavailable to give emotional support to your partner, by not keeping promises you've made, or by getting into arguments when you were upset about problems unrelated to your partner. You might have damaged your relationship with your children by being absent for their activities because you were too involved with your addiction, by not spending time with them, by breaking promises, or by yelling at them. You've probably also damaged your relationship with friends, other family members, and colleagues or fellow workers.

## Exercise 1:   Damage to Relationships.

In the space provided below, list your relationships that have been damaged by your chemical use. Under each one, give some specific examples that illustrate how you have damaged that relationship. If you have trouble completing this exercise, go back to Chapter One (Secrets and Lies). This review will most likely refresh your memory:

_____

_____

_____

_____

_____

_____

## Example:

My wife, Nancy:

    a.  I wasted family money on cocaine, then I got angry with her when she asked me about it.

    b.  During her pregnancy, when she most needed my emotional support, I was too focused on cocaine.

    c.  I lied to her about why I was coming home late.

1. _____

    a. _____

    b. _____

    c. _____

    d. _____

    e. _____

2. _____

    a. _____

    b. _____

    c. _____

    d. _____

    e. _____

3. _____

    a. _____

    b. _____

    c. _____

    d. _____

    e. _____

4. _____

    a. _____

    b. _____

    c. _____

    d. _____

    e. _____

5. _____

    a. _____

    b. _____

    c. _____

    d. _____

    e. _____

## Exercise 2: Damage to My Career

In the space below, describe any ways that you have damaged your career because of your chemical use.

_____

_____

_____

_____

_____

_____

_____

_____

_____

# Soul Damage

Failure to nurture yourself contributes to the pain and feelings of despair felt by an addict. When you can't nurture yourself, you also can't feel connected to anyone.

Spiritual traditions typically teach about the sacredness of activities based on values that respect the soul in everyone. Every relationship is sacred but addict behavior moves you away from that sacredness and self respect.

All addicts lie to somebody, and all addicts lie to themselves. Continual lying hurts all relationships; the relationship that is damaged most of all is your relationship with yourself. The more you damage the relationship with yourself through lying and other destructive behaviors, the more you lose sight of your inner self, your authentic self, your soul. Loss to the soul takes away the most important component of internal motivation. Without that motivation, there is little that keeps the addict from believing there is any way to reduce pain other than drug use.

Now is the time to be really honest with yourself. It is time to admit how your use of alcohol or other drugs has damaged your soul.

## Exercise 3:   Soul Damage

In the space provided below, list the ways you have damaged your soul by engaging in behaviors that have led to destruction of important relationships in your life. How have you betrayed your own value system? How has your drug use interfered with your ability to nurture yourself or be connected to others?

_____

_____

_____

_____

_____

_____

_____

_____

_____

# Completing a Damage-Control Plan

If you have worked through the previous exercises and those in the preceding chapters, you undoubtedly have a pretty good idea of the damage that drug-related behaviors have inflicted on you and others. Congratulations! You have already taken the first step on the path to recovery, which is to recognize that your life has become unmanageable and that, until now, you have been powerless to change it.

You might be asking, "How do I begin to change?" Until now, you have lived by a set of beliefs that have led you to behave in certain ways. To summarize, some of these beliefs and actions have been:

1. No one knows or will know. Therefore, I must operate in secrecy.

2. I can change my behavior by myself. I can always figure out or force a way to handle problems. I work best alone. Therefore, I must isolate myself from others. I can't tell anyone the whole story about myself.

3. I have not hurt others or myself by what I have done. Therefore, I can continue with my grandiosity, my double life, and living in chaos.

To recover, you need to change both your beliefs and your actions. Here are a healthier set of beliefs and their corresponding actions:

1. There are no secrets. Therefore, I must make a full disclosure.

2. I am powerless to change without the help of others. I need contact with and the help of others. Therefore, I must create support networks. I must tell my whole story to trustworthy people.

3. I have repeatedly caused damage to myself and others. Therefore, I must begin to behave with integrity. I must exercise humility and embrace my mistakes and needs. I have a damage-control plan, and I seek the help of others.

## Exercise 4:   My Attempts to Control My Drug Use

Using your previous beliefs and ways of acting on them, list five examples of changes you made in your life in an effort to control your behavior around your drug use or to make your life different. Include such examples as changing jobs, moving, and leaving relationships.

1. _____
2. _____
3. _____
4. _____
5. _____

What were some of the beliefs that led you to attempt to change your life?

1. _____
2. _____
3. _____
4. _____
5. _____

List five steps you have taken, since you have begun this program, that have led or that will lead to your new way of thinking and acting. Don't forget the effort you have put into this workbook:

1. _____
2. _____
3. _____
4. _____
5. _____

It is undoubtedly easier to change your behavior than your beliefs. It will most likely take you quite some time before you really believe that you can change in basic ways, before you really believe you can trust other people. This is normal. Two relevant slogans in the 12-Step Program of Alcoholics Anonymous (AA) are: "Act 'as if,'" and "Walk the walk." When you begin to behave differently, people will treat you differently. If you behave with integrity and respect, people will begin to treat you as a person of integrity who is to be respected. Soon you will begin to believe that you are a person of integrity. Changed behaviors lead to changed beliefs. So even if you secretly believe you are slime, you should act "as if" you are an authentic person who is acting with integrity. Move forward with the process, and eventually your inner feelings will change.

Now it is time to make a written damage control plan. First, make a list of your current problems. Refer to your list in Chapter One if you run out of ideas. This time, however, focus only on your *current* problems, in particular the ones that have been caused by your addictive behavior. These may be in the categories of health problems, relationship problems, job problems, legal problems, or financial problems.

## Current Problem List

1. _____

_____

2. _____

_____

3. _____

_____

4. _____

_____

5. _____

_____

6. _____

_____

7. _____

_____

8. _____

_____

On the pages that follow, you will find forms that allow you to think logically and in an organized way through each of the problems you have just listed. Use one form per problem. You will find that this way of thinking through problems is not only helpful now, at the beginning of your recovery when things are chaotic and overwhelming, but that you also can use it on an ongoing basis as normal life difficulties arise.

For each problem, write the following:

*Best possible outcome:* What would be the best result of any actions you might take or plan you might devise?

*Minimal acceptable outcome:* What is the minimal result that is acceptable?

*Possible solutions:* Brainstorm with your support system and list all the solutions that everyone came up with, no matter how far fetched.

*Best solution:* From all the possible solutions, write down the best one or a combination of ideas.

*Action steps with target dates:* What concrete actions do you need to take? By what date will you take them?

*Support needed:* What do you need in order to take these steps, and who do you need to help you?

# Damage-Control Worksheet

Problem:

_____

_____

_____

_____

_____

Best Possible Outcome:

_____

_____

_____

_____

_____

Minimum Acceptable Outcome:

_____

_____

_____

_____

_____

Possible Solutions:

1. _____

_____

2. _____

_____

3. _____

_____

4. _____

_____

5. _____

_____

6. _____

_____

7. _____

_____

8. _____

_____

9. _____

_____

10. _____

_____

Best Possible Solutions:

_____

_____

_____

_____

_____

Action Steps:

1. _____

_____

Date taken by: _____

2. _____

_____

Date taken by: _____

3. _____

_____

Date taken by: _____

4. _____

_____

Date taken by: _____

5. _____

_____

Date taken by: _____

Support Needed:

_____

_____

_____

_____

_____

# Damage-Control Worksheet

Problem:

_____

_____

_____

_____

_____

Best Possible Outcome:

_____

_____

_____

_____

_____

Minimum Acceptable Outcome:

_____

_____

_____

_____

_____

Possible Solutions:

1. _____

_____

2. _____

_____

3. _____

_____

4. _____

5. _____

6. _____

7. _____

8. _____

9. _____

10. _____

Best Possible Solutions:

_____

_____

_____

_____

_____

Action Steps:

1. _____

Date taken by: _____

2. _____

Date taken by: _____

3. _____

_____

Date taken by: _____

4. _____

_____

Date taken by: _____

5. _____

_____

Date taken by: _____

Support needed

_____

_____

_____

_____

_____

_____

# Damage-Control Worksheet

Problem:

_____

_____

_____

_____

_____

Best Possible Outcome:

_____

_____

_____

_____

_____

Minimum Acceptable Outcome:

_____

_____

_____

_____

_____

Possible Solutions:

1. _____

_____

2. _____

_____

3. _____

_____

4. _____

_____

5. _____

_____

6. _____

_____

7. _____

_____

8. _____

_____

9. _____

_____

10. _____

_____

Best Possible Solutions:

_____

_____

_____

_____

_____

Action Steps:

1. _____

_____

Date taken by: _____

2. _____

_____

Date taken by: _____

3. _____

_____

Date taken by: _____

4. _____

_____

Date taken by: _____

5. _____

_____

Date taken by: _____

Support Needed:

_____

_____

_____

_____

_____

_____

# Damage-Control Worksheet

Problem:

_____

_____

_____

_____

_____

Best Possible Outcome:

_____

_____

_____

_____

_____

Minimum Acceptable Outcome:

_____

_____

_____

_____

_____

Possible Solutions:

1. _____

_____

2. _____

_____

3. _____

_____

4. _____

_____

5. _____

_____

6. _____

_____

7. _____

_____

8. _____

_____

9. _____

_____

10. _____

_____

Best Possible Solutions:

_____

_____

_____

_____

_____

Action Steps:

1. _____

_____

Date taken by: _____

2. _____

_____

Date taken by: _____

3. _____

_____

Date taken by: _____

4. _____

_____

Date taken by: _____

5. _____

_____

Date taken by: _____

Support Needed:

_____

_____

_____

_____

_____

_____

# Damage by Disclosure—and by Nondisclosure

Because addicts lie, most addicts have secrets. Secrets create walls between people, often require additional lies to protect the secrets, and delay recovery. Long ago, the founders of AA recognized the importance of honesty in recovery; today, rigorous honesty is still a cornerstone of their twelve step recovery plan.

When you think about disclosing your secrets, a motion picture may flash through your head. In it, your spouse or partner is furious upon hearing your disclosure—and leaves you. Your friend, having heard your truth, decides you are too slimy to continue the friendship. Your kids no longer respect you. Your boss fires you. When you picture such outcomes, you may be naturally reluctant to say anything to anyone.

There is a right way and a right time to disclose, and there are right and wrong people to disclose to. Many chemically dependent people act out sexually while they are under the influence, so you might have sexual secrets to disclose. You might also have secrets involving lies about the money you spent on your addiction, the places you visited, illegal activities in which you participated in connection with your addiction, difficulties you have had at work, and so on. None of these are easy to disclose, but it will be worse for you if your partner finds out about them from someone else. The following sections summarize the statements of some recovering addicts and their partners or spouses about their experience with disclosure, what worked well for them and what didn't, and what they would recommend to others. You can read about their experience in greater detail in our book *Disclosing Secrets: What, to Whom, and How Much to Reveal.*

## What Are My Secrets?

Before deciding how much, to whom, how, and when to disclose, you need to give thought again to your secrets. Have you lied to your spouse about where you've been spending a lot of your time? Have you stuffed away your anger or resentment because you hate conflict, and then used your drug of choice in an effort to control your anger? Have you avoided talking about the emotional baggage in your relationship because it seems too heavy to carry around, only to find yourself carrying a heavier load due to all your lies surrounding your drug use? Do you have large gambling debts? Have you stolen money from your workplace? Do you have a secret hoard of money from drug dealing? Have you borrowed from your children's college fund to pay for your drugs? Have you been warned by your boss that after one more absence you'll be fired? Are you having extramarital sex as part of your drug use? Are you HIV positive as a result of drug use or unprotected sex with other partners? Have you told so many lies that you don't know when you are lying or telling the truth?

## Exercise 5:   My Secrets

Make a list of all the secrets you are keeping related to your drug activities. Be specific. If it would make you feel more comfortable, write the list in your private journal where it is less likely to seen by others. Leave some space below each item, as you will be adding more material later in this chapter.

1. _____

_____

_____

_____

_____

_____

2. _____

_____

_____

_____

_____

_____

3. _____

_____

_____

_____

_____

_____

4. _____
_____
_____
_____
_____
_____

5. _____
_____
_____
_____
_____
_____

6. _____
_____
_____
_____
_____
_____
_____
_____

7. _____
_____
_____
_____
_____

8. _____
_____
_____
_____
_____
_____

Please take a few minutes to review your secrets list in Chapter One. Are there differences between the lists? To what do you attribute those differences? If you need to make any changes to the list above based on your review, do so now.

_____

_____

_____

_____

_____

_____

# To Whom Should I Disclose?

Brandon was a recovering cocaine addict with two years' recovery when he began a new job as associate marketing director of a large psychiatric hospital. Like the majority of cocaine addicts, he had also been compulsively sexual during his drug-using days, visiting prostitutes and engaging in cocaine-sex binges. He considered those days to be "ancient history," and he was now very active in Cocaine Anonymous and Sex Addicts Anonymous. An outgoing and energetic person, he was doing very well in his job when he decided that "rigorous honesty" demanded that he disclose his addiction history to his boss. Within two weeks, he was told that he was being let go because sufficient funds were no longer available for his position.

Being honest does not mean telling everything to everyone. Depending on the nature of the disclosure, there are certain people who do need to know.

The _therapist or counselor_ you are seeing for your addiction clearly needs to know everything in order to be able to help you. It is natural to balk at first about revealing the worst things about yourself; after all, you want your therapist to like you. You feel shame at the thought of revealing yourself. Remind yourself that your therapist is used to hearing disclosures similar to yours—and undoubtedly worse ones. He or she is there specifically to help you deal with the consequences of your acts and to help you learn how to cope more successfully with life. In order to do this, your therapist has to know everything you have done.

*Your spouse or significant other* also needs to know. A healthy, intimate relationship requires open sharing between two people. If you are feeling shame about your behavior and have erected a wall between you and your partner in order to hide the secret, there is no way you can have real intimacy.

A second reason to disclose to your partner is that he or she has been directly affected by your actions. If you have acquired a sexually transmitted disease, have spent family money, are about to lose your job, or are in legal trouble, your partner's life is about to change, and he or she has the right to know. With this information, your partner is now in a position to make some choices, such as whether or not to stay in the relationship and whether or not to continue to be sexual with you.

A third reason your partner needs to know is for his or her own recovery. Addiction is crazy-making for the people around the addict. Again and again, partners are asked to believe what the addict says rather than what their gut is telling them. He says, "I had to work late," when he was in fact at his dealer's house. He says, "That woman you saw me with was just a client," when she was in fact a partner in an affair. He says, "If you weren't such a lousy house-keeper, I wouldn't have to drink so much." The partner comes to believe that she is defective and ineffective, that her gut feelings are unreliable, that she caused the problem, and that if she can only figure out the right thing to do, she can solve it. Knowing the truth, and recognizing that addiction is a family disease, can lead partners to seek help for themselves. Your spouse or partner needs support in coping with your disclosure and in determining how to respond to it. An excellent source of support is Al-Anon, a twelve-step program for families and friends of alcoholics (and, these days, of drug addicts). Counseling can be very beneficial as well.

*Your twelve-step sponsor* also needs to know everything. This is a person in the program who has taken on the job of mentoring you in your recovery. Sponsors do this as part of their own recovery. In Chapter 9 we will explain their role in more detail. For now, it's important that you know that, like your counselor, your sponsor needs all the information about your addiction in order to effectively direct you in your recovery. An addict himself, your sponsor truly understands and can hear you out without being judgmental.

*Your children* have a need to know about matters that affect them, in age-appropriate ways. Children notice everything around them, but they also pick up cues about what to ask. If certain subjects are not discussed in the home, the children learn to stay silent. It is much healthier for them to receive explanations. For example, if you are often out in the evenings attending twelve-step meetings, you can tell your five year old, "I got into some bad habits that made it harder for me to be a good parent to you. I was paying too much attention to other things. I am now being helped each evening, and because of the help, I'll be able to do a much better job." An adolescent will, of course, need a more specific explanation.

*Your doctor* needs to know things you are doing that affect your health. It is possible to diagnose chronic excessive drinking on the basis of objective data (elevated blood pressure, abnormal liver function tests, enlarged red blood cells, and increased uric acid levels in the blood). It is hard to hide a two-pack per day smoking addiction because of the odor of stale smoke that quickly fills the examining room. But other drug use can be hidden for longer. Your physician's job is to keep you healthy and to solve your medical problems, but it is hard to do so if you are lying about what you are putting into your body.

*Other relatives, employer, and friends*: Disclose to these people on a need-to-know basis. If your drug use has had a direct impact on them, then tell them about your behaviors. Before doing so, it is wise to consult your sponsor. If you are considering disclosing to your in-laws or to friends who are your partner's friends as well, discuss this with your partner or spouse. Think about your motive for disclosure, and consider the possible consequences and the most likely outcome.

## Exercise 6:  Who to Tell

Go back to your list of secrets in Exercise 5. Below each secret, write down the following:

(a)     The names of the person(s) who need to hear this secret.

(b)     The benefit(s) of disclosing to each person.

# How Much Should I Disclose?

Some addicts are so fearful of the consequences of telling that they disclose as little as possible. If they think the listener already knows something, they confess only to that. Or else they reveal only the smallest mistake they made, leaving the really bad stuff for later. On the other hand, some addicts are so tired of the burden of secrets and lies that they reveal every single misdeed, in great detail, completely overwhelming the listener.

Neither of these methods is desirable. What works best is to make a list of all your secrets and initially disclose the broad outlines of each. Don't leave out anything important! But you also don't need to include any details that your spouse or partner may later regret hearing. This is particularly true when the disclosure includes sexual behaviors. In such a case, you don't need to disclose how many times, what exactly you did in bed, and so forth. (At some later time, if your partner has additional questions, it is important that they be answered, but we are talking about planning your initial disclosure.) What does matter, however, is to not leave out anything important.

> Lance and Linda, parents of two young children, had not had a vacation for three years because Lance's income was just enough to cover their living expenses. One day, Linda found a check stub that Lance had carefully hidden under the seat of his car. It showed that a year ago he'd gotten a $100 per week raise, but he had been skimming the $100 off each paycheck. Linda confronted Lance with the evidence the moment he returned from visiting Bob next door. Angry that Linda had been snooping in his car, Lance starting deflecting the blame by focusing on her attention to their children instead of to him. At first he made up lies about spending the money on fixing the car. When she said "prove it," he blurted out, "Okay! Okay! If you must know, I can't stand my life with you. You let those kids rule the house. I can't stand it. Do you want to know what I've been doing with that money? I've been buying cocaine for myself and a couple of friends at work who appreciate my talents."

> Linda couldn't believe that Lance had sacrificed the family for his drug habit or that he had said such horrible things about how she cared for their children. She realized that he'd repeatedly lied to her, and she wondered if her trust in him could be restored. She began to wonder aloud if she'd be better off without Lance. When the possibility of actually losing Linda and their children became real to him, Lance begged for another chance. He agreed to attend church on a regular basis with Linda and the kids, and he started helping more with things around the house. He became involved in Cocaine Anonymous on a regular basis, and he stopped skimming off part of his paycheck. After three months, Linda was convinced that Lance was serious about his recovery and about their relationship. She was beginning to trust him again.

One evening, there was a knock on the door. It was the police, there to arrest Lance for having sold cocaine. Although he was no longer selling it, one of his former customers had just been arrested for possession and had given the police Lance's name.

Linda was devastated. Not only was her husband apparently headed for prison, but when he had disclosed his cocaine addiction to her he had failed to reveal the most important part—that he'd been a dealer as well. He had continued to withhold this information from her during the three months that he had insisted he was being honest. She decided she could never trust him again and was not interested in waiting for him to get out of prison. She divorced him.

What is particularly destructive to relationships is staggered disclosure—revealing only the most acceptable secrets at first, and leaving the worst for later. We strongly recommend giving the main elements of all your secrets the first time around.

# When Should I Disclose?

Many addicts don't really have a choice about the timing of disclosure. When someone repeatedly drinks excessively, this is usually evident to his wife and friends. If someone is arrested for drug possession or dealing, again, the family will immediately learn what's going on. But in other cases the addict has successfully hidden the addiction, so he or she does have the option of when to reveal it. Or the spouse has learned about part of the addiction but doesn't know about the rest of it.

Addicts in early recovery are often advised not to disclose anything until they have had some time in recovery and have thoroughly discussed it with their sponsor and their group. It is also a good idea to be sure that the spouse or partner has some support so they will be able to debrief and get help from a counselor or friend. These are good suggestions. Unfortunately, all too often they are used as an excuse for delaying disclosure far longer than it should be. Disclosure is an uncomfortable process. It is bound to cause shame for the addict and pain for the spouse or partner, and it potentially leads to adverse consequences, such as divorce or being fired. No wonder the addict is inclined to put it off! Getting more time in recovery is a great excuse to do so.

One unfortunate consequence of delaying disclosure is that the secret keeping and the lying continue, and new lies are necessary. How will you explain your time away from home for meetings? How about the phone calls you and your sponsor are now exchanging? The longer you lie to your partner, the worse it will be when you finally do disclose. And if your partner learns about your addiction before you get around to disclosing—and this gets increasingly likely with time—your partner will be even more upset.

*Preparing for disclosure needs to be a priority in early recovery.* Talk with your counselor, your group, and your sponsor. Arrange for support for your partner and then proceed with disclosure, preferably in the setting of a counseling session.

# Completing a Disclosure Plan

Now is a good time for you to prepare a disclosure plan. The following disclosure plan outline is from *Facing the Shadow* by Patrick Carnes (Gentle Path Press, 2001). We recommend that you complete it and then review it with your therapist, sponsor, and group.

## Exercise 7:   Filling Out a Disclosure Plan

List ten persons, more or less, to whom you need to disclose at least some facts about your drug and alcohol addiction. These may include your therapist, sponsor, partner, employer, children, other relatives, friends, and others. After each, be specific about what you wish to tell and what your goal is in telling them. Review your excuses to use, problems list, lies from Chapter One (Exercises 3, 4, 5), and your secrets list earlier in this chapter to be sure you are covering all the topics you need to disclose. Record when you will do this, with whom, and where you intend to get support.

1. Person:_____

   Material to be disclosed:_____

   _____

   _____

Goal:_____

Timing:_____

Support from:_____

2. Person:_____

   Material to be disclosed:_____

   _____

   _____

   Goal:_____

   Timing:_____

   Support from:_____

3. Person:_____

   Material to be disclosed:_____

   _____

   _____

   Goal:_____

   Timing:_____

   Support from:_____

4. Person:_____

   Material to be disclosed:_____

   _____

   _____

   Goal:_____

   Timing:_____

   Support from:_____

5. Person:_____

   Material to be disclosed:_____

   _____

   _____

Goal:_____

Timing:_____

Support from:_____

6. Person:_____

   Material to be disclosed:_____

   _____

   _____

   Goal:_____

   Timing:_____

   Support from:_____

7. Person:_____

   Material to be disclosed:_____

   _____

   _____

   Goal:_____

   Timing:_____

   Support from:_____

8. Person:_____

   Material to be disclosed:_____

   _____

   _____

   Goal:_____

   Timing:_____

   Support from:_____

9. Person:_____

   Material to be disclosed:_____

   _____

   _____

Goal:_____     _____

Timing:_____

Support from:_____

10.  Person:_____

Material to be disclosed:_____

_____

_____

Goal:_____

Timing:_____

Support from:_____

# Developing a Press Release

Developing a statement to use when someone you don't know suddenly asks about your addiction is very helpful. Your therapist and sponsor can provide a great deal of help in creating a short statement that is truthful but that allows for common sense and privacy. Your spouse or partner needs to know and agree on what is said. Sometimes it is helpful for your children to have something they can say. This will help keep everyone from getting caught up in the shame of the disease. Remember that some information about your addiction is private, especially to those outside your primary relationships. You can refuse to give any more information, no matter how much you are asked.

As we continue our work in the next chapter, we'll focus on establishing accountability with ourselves and important people in our lives, learning to develop empathy for the victims of our behavior, and achieving peace and serenity through forgiveness.

# CHAPTER SEVEN: Healing Relationships through Accountability

**accountable** adj. *obliged to account for one's acts, responsible*

During your active addiction days, did you ever contemplate—or actually carry out—a "geographic cure?" By this, we mean that, when a person finds himself in enough difficulties in one job, or in one city, or in one relationship, his solution is to relocate and start all over. It is always tempting to leave behind the mess you have created rather than experience the pain, shame, and accountability involved in staying put and solving the mess. Unfortunately, this rarely works; the one thing you have taken with you to your new location is *you*, and you are likely to replicate your problems wherever you go.

When you have severely damaged your relationships, whether with your partner, your children, or your friends, it is equally tempting to start anew. It takes courage to work through the distrust, resentments, pain, anger, and other negative feelings that other people feel in response to your addiction. "Half measures availed us not," said the early members of AA. Rebuilding your marriage and other relationships will not work if you are on the fence, ready to flee if the work seems too hard. Your chances of success will be far greater if you recommit to your relationships and are determined to do your best to undo the damage and make them stronger than ever.

# Establishing Agreements for Accountability

When your life was centered on drinking and drugging, you were probably irresponsible on more than one occasion. You most likely made promises to your partner, your children, and your boss, and then broke them. You mouthed commitments but never took them seriously. You did not feel accountable to anyone. This is why, now that you have seriously committed to your recovery and to your relationships, it is time to put accountability in your life. Eventually, the most important person to whom you will be accountable is yourself. You will avoid self-destructive behaviors even if no one else will find out about them, because *you* will know about your behavior, and because you recognize that this behavior is harmful to you and others.

At the beginning, however, you need the help of other people to keep you on the straight and narrow. The most important is your sponsor, the person who has committed to helping you on a twenty-four-hour basis to recover. Develop a plan with your sponsor on ways you can be accountable to him or her. Here are some suggestions for possible actions; your final agreement will vary depending on the people involved:

- Agree that you will phone your sponsor at least once a day and tell him how you are feeling. If you get comfortable with making these routine calls, it will be that much easier for you to phone your sponsor urgently if you are on the verge of drinking or using again.

- Agree that if you must be in a place where you feel unsafe—for example, your cousin's wedding where there will be drinking—you will "bookend" the event. This means you will phone the sponsor at the beginning of the event and again at the end.

- Agree to attend a certain number of twelve-step meetings per week, and discuss each meeting afterwards with your sponsor. Commonly at the very beginning of recovery, addicts commit to "90 in 90," that is, attending 90 meetings in 90 days.

- Agree that if you have a slip, you will immediately report it to your sponsor.

## Exercise 1:  My Accountability Plan

After you have discussed your accountability with your sponsor, write a list of what you have agreed to:

1. _____

2. _____

3. _____

If you wish to rebuild your relationship with your spouse or partner, it is crucial that you be accountable to him/her. Below are some agreements you might make with your partner:

- Keep your promises. If you promise to be somewhere or do something, follow through.

- Account for your time. If you are going to be late, call and explain why.

- If secret spending was an issue, agree to review your expenditures with your partner.

- Discuss with your partner how much she wants to know about any relapses, slips, and near-slips. Your sponsor and twelve-step group need to be the primary recipients of this information, but your spouse may want to know about activities that directly impact your relationship.

**Caution**: In your efforts to be accountable to your spouse or partner, *do not make them your parent equivalent*. For example, you might think it's a good idea to have your spouse hold on to all the money and dole out to you only what you need for the day, so that you will not be tempted to spend it on drugs. Forget it! This is a disaster for most couples who use money issues in an attempt to gain control in a relationship. Instead, get an accountability partner (someone you can trust to help you be accountable but who isn't in a love relationship with you.) Converting your equal partnership into a parent-child situation can be very harmful for the relationship. Inevitably you will feel resentful and want to rebel, while your partner is likely to become angry and judgmental.

With accountability issues, your personal agenda is paramount. It is important to be accountable for your time and for your own sobriety. If you are being accountable because you want to remain in recovery *and* rebuild trust, you are on the right track. If you call home to check in because you adore your partner and want to let her know it, calling will feel good and enhance your recovery. If you are calling because you are scared and don't want your partner to be suspicious, look out. Pretty soon, you will be resentful and your partner will sense the resentment and will probably start acting as if she doesn't trust you again, making it harder to feel good about the relationship. Clean up your personal agenda to reflect your recovery first. If you are being honest with yourself about your actions—really honest—the rebuilding will be a natural result of that effort.

Another person to whom you need to be accountable is your counselor. Your agreement might include keeping all your appointments, being honest about any slips or temptations, and following through on homework assignments.

# Cost of My Addiction

If, in your Current Problems List, you had nothing related to how much you have spent on your drugs, then you are an exception. The direct costs of addiction are usually very high for everyone who has an addiction. Even if you use drugs only occasionally, you have probably spent more than you planned.

## Exercise 2: What Has It Cost Me?

Seeing how much you have spent in black and white (or red) helps you to know not only how it is a problem, but that what you have spent could have been used better elsewhere. This exercise is for that purpose. You don't have to be compulsive in listing costs, as good estimates are more than adequate to provide you with the result you need. Here is a general ledger for completing the financial analysis. Complete this project for the past year, and then repeat it for at least the last five years of your substance use. You may use your journal or add columns on this ledger.

# Total estimate of resources spent on my habit:

**Direct Expenses Estimates**

Purchase price of my substance. _____

Expenses obtaining substance (e.g., for transportation, phone, computer time). _____

Money lost by selling my possessions to obtain money for drugs. _____

Spending while "under the influence". (going to bars or clubs, travel, special clothes or paraphernalia, money for entertainment while using, motels, Internet, etc.) _____

Money spent on legal fees, fines, and probation. _____

Money spent on therapy or previous rehabilitation efforts. _____

**Total of direct expenses:** _____

**Indirect Expenses Estimates**

Lost wages and earnings. _____

Money diverted for drug use from my employers, family, and other people. Include theft of property. _____

Medical expenses, including over-the-counter drugs for treating hangovers or other drug effects. _____

Cost of therapy and drug treatment (Rehab.). _____

Cost of accidents associated with substance use. _____

Lost or damaged property associated with use. _____

Costs associated with ending marriages or business ventures with other partners. _____

Any other legal expenses and court fees (such as hiring a lawyer in an attempt to save my job or professional license). _____

Other Expenses. _____

Total of direct expenses: _____

Add the total of direct expenses: _____

# Grand total. _____

    You might find it interesting to calculate your average annual expenses during the past five years.

    Now, reflect on the results of your financial analysis. What conclusion or thoughts come to mind as you ponder the results? How do you weigh the benefits of drug use against these costs? What would you do with this money if it were available to you today? What did your family, business, or others give up because you spent these resources on your drugs? Record your thoughts here:

_____
_____
_____
_____
_____
_____

Before you leave this section, record five examples of your denial or minimization regarding your spending associated with substance use:

(*Example:* I could never get my credit card balances paid down. I never saw this as a result of spending on my substance of choice until now.)

1. _____
_____

2. _____
_____

3. _____
_____

4. _____
_____

5. _____
_____

# Victim Empathy

It is important for you to begin to think about those you have victimized with your behavior. You have not really addressed one of the most costly components of your addiction until you do. Remember, anyone touched by your drug use is a victim—some more than others.

Recovery is about never again having victims.

One way to achieve this is to learn what it feels like to be a victim, to walk a mile in the victim's moccasins. Have you ever identified with a character in a movie or a book? If you did, it was probably because you recognized what the character was feeling because you have experienced that same feeling on some level as well. Understanding how someone else feels is called *empathy*. Understanding how victims feel is called *victim empathy*. If you have become immune to feelings in an effort to stay in denial about the seriousness of your behavior, it may take you a while to really begin to let in the feelings of empathy.

Some addicts enjoy inflicting pain on other people because it makes them feel powerful: The addict can make someone else have feelings he doesn't want to have. Other addicts (for example, a crack addict who steals his mother's jewelry, sells it, and buys more crack) choose not to accept that their behavior causes emotional, spiritual, and/or physical pain to their victims.

Take a moment to think about something that happened to you in the past that was hurtful, unpleasant, or saddening. Who empathized with you? How did you know they understood how you felt? Think about how those around you have felt as a result of your behavior.

For you to develop empathy, you must learn to feel *and accept* your own powerlessness. Accepting it means being willing to know it exists and to feel it. When you accept your feelings of fear, powerlessness, and inadequacy, you will be able to feel the pain of others. When you accept your painful feelings, you will more fully experience joy and happiness, too. You can only empathize with feelings you are willing to experience yourself. If you are unwilling to feel shame, you can't empathize with someone else's shame.

Another way to start learning empathy is to imagine a time when you felt terrible. It may have been when you were beaten up as a child, got arrested for a DUI, or went bankrupt. Perhaps you were sexually or physically victimized when you were young. Whatever it was, allow yourself to remember the intensity of those feelings. Still another way is to imagine you are a victim of a crime or of someone else acting out on you. Think about the old feelings you had and allow them to become stronger. Victims feel intensely. No matter how intensely painful, or sorrowful, or depressed you are about your behavior as an addict, your victims felt and feel worse.

Feeling sad for someone else's misfortune is a form of empathy; feeling sorry for yourself is self-pity. Self-pity keeps you from looking at the effects of your behaviors on others. It enables you to continue your addictive behavior. Self-pity does not help you change; it encourages you to blame others for your misfortunes, mistakes, using, acting out, and consequences. When you're wrapped up in self-pity, you focus on what you don't like and how everyone else is better off than you. You use it to feed your anger and greed instead of making productive changes.

Disgust about your drug use is an appropriate and realistic feeling for an addict. Being disgusted with the pain you have caused and the people you have affected is a step in the right direction. But, it works only when you can *use this feeling to motivate yourself to change.* Without a commitment to change, being disgusted with yourself is another form of self-pity, and that feeling is frequently used as a reason to relapse.

When you are able to have empathy for your victim's pain, acknowledge what you have done that has contributed to their feelings. The more you are able to see and acknowledge your victim's feelings, the quicker she or he will be able to accept your amends and move toward forgiveness.

# Forgiveness Takes Time

What comes to mind when you consider the role of forgiveness in your life? Most likely you are thinking, "Will my partner ever forgive me for the misery I've caused her?" Perhaps even, "Will the person I injured when I was driving drunk ever forgive me?" It may take you a while to realize that you, too, need to forgive. Undoubtedly there are people in your life who have hurt you. These might include an alcoholic father who abused you physically or emotionally, a mother who was so focused on your alcoholic father that she never had time for you, an adult who sexually abused you, a spouse who was controlling and judgmental. And don't forget that you need to forgive yourself—for the mess you have created in your life, for the pain you have caused yourself and others, for your negative thoughts and feelings about your worthlessness. You can probably add other items to this list.

What's the big deal about forgiveness? It is important because, in order to get on with your life, you need to forgive those who have hurt you. Otherwise the resentments you feel about the wrong done to you will continue to eat away at you and prevent you from achieving serenity in your recovery. The main purpose of forgiving is to bring peace to yourself, not to absolve the other person of his wrongdoing. Forgiving is healing for the forgiver.

In his excellent book *Forgive and Forget: Healing the Hurts We Don't Deserve*, Lewis B. Smedes describes what forgiveness is *not*. First, forgiving is not forgetting. By forgiving someone, you do not forget the hurtful acts. You need to forgive precisely because you have not forgotten what someone did; your memory keeps the pain alive long after the actual wrongdoing is past. Because forgiving is healing, it will make it easier to forget. But it is not necessary to forget the past in order to forgive. What forgiving will accomplish is to heal the pain of the past.

Second, forgiving is not excusing. Excusing is the opposite of forgiving. You excuse a person when you believe he was not to blame for the wrong he did; you forgive him because you believe that he was to blame. This is why excusing is easy, but forgiving is hard.

Finally, forgiving is not tolerating. You can forgive someone without tolerating what he did. You can forgive your father for his years of constantly demeaning and insulting you, without being willing to tolerate this behavior in the future. This might require that you not have an ongoing relationship with him. Forgiveness does not imply acceptance of the behavior in the past or future.

What, then, is forgiveness? Forgiveness is healing yourself of the painful memories of the past. This is a slow process that may take years. It involves several steps.

# Steps to Forgiving

1. Recognize that a wrong has been done to you. Instead of making excuses, acknowledge that this person's behavior was inexcusable and that he behaved in ways that caused you a great deal of pain.

2. Recognize that you have strong feelings about the wrong that was done to you; feel those feelings, which undoubtedly include anger and hate.

3. Share your strong feelings with others. It would be ideal to confront the responsible person and tell him directly how you feel about what he did, but often this is not possible—he may be unavailable or no longer alive, or he may have made it clear he is not interested in your feelings. Or you may be too fearful of his reaction to risk direct confrontation. In either case, sharing with your support group or therapist will allow you to express your emotions about the situation. This is preferable to swallowing them

and turning them into depression, turning them into aggression, or drinking or using over them.

4.  Understand the other person's vulnerabilities that may have led him to hurt you. Your parents may themselves have had difficult childhoods. Your spouse or partner may have been overwhelmed by a full-time job combined with all the parenting responsibilities. And so forth. This is not an attempt to excuse the person's behavior, but rather to understand that he too is a flawed human being.

5.  Recognize your role in the other person's hurtful behavior. Your spouse's demanding, controlling, judgmental, and critical stance may have resulted from months or years of feeling powerless, angry, and frustrated because of your lies, your failures to keep commitments, and other problems related to your addiction. Accepting your share of responsibility for your pain will help you forgive the other person.

6.  Determine what role you want from the other person in the future: Do you want an ongoing relationship? If not, then all you can do is heal your bitterness toward him and wish him well. You cannot change the facts of the person's past actions, but you can divorce the past from how you feel about him. If he is still causing pain to others, you can say a prayer for him and hope that a higher power will eventually show him the way toward recovery. Forgiving him will give you a sense of peace and allow you to get on with your life.

7.  If you and the other person are interested in salvaging the relationship, forgiving him or her will be easiest if the other person is remorseful and asks for forgiveness.

## Steps to Asking for Forgiveness

Asking forgiveness is not just saying some words. Just like forgiving someone else, being worthy of forgiveness is a process. Its key element is remorse. Here is how it can be done:

1.  Recognize that your actions were hurtful and unfair.
2.  Feel the pain you caused the other person, and feel guilt about what you did.
3.  Tell the other person what actions you are asking forgiveness for.
4.  Describe to the other person the feeling you recognize he or she felt as a result of your hurtful actions.
5.  Ask to be forgiven.

6. Commit to not hurting the person in this way again.

As we have said before, just promising not to do something is not enough; you need to follow up your words with action steps (see the section on Establishing Agreements for Accountability).

In your early addiction recovery, you have two tasks regarding forgiveness:

1. Identify the people whom you have hurt and from whom you wish forgiveness, and then walk through the steps that will make it easier for you to be forgiven.

2. Identify those people that you need to forgive, and work toward forgiving them.

## Exercise 3:   Forgiveness

Awareness is the first step in the forgiveness process. Make two lists below. The first is of those people you can think of whom you need to forgive (Don't forget yourself!), and the second is of people you have hurt and from whom you want to ask forgiveness. Next to each person, list one thing that will change if you forgive them or if they forgive you.

**People to forgive**

1. _____
2. _____
3. _____
4. _____
5. _____
6. _____
7. _____
8. _____
9. _____
10. _____

**People from whom to ask for forgiveness**

1. _____
2. _____
3. _____
4. _____
5. _____
6. _____
7. _____
8. _____
9. _____
10. _____

# Rebuilding Trust

Ruthann complained to her AA friends, "I'm getting really tired of Rick's suspicions. I've seen him searching the places in the house where I used to hide my bottles. When we're at parties, he never leaves me alone, and if he sees me drinking some ginger ale, he sniffs the glass to make sure I haven't spiked it. He grills me about which friends I see, and he wants a detailed report on every AA meeting I attend, like he doesn't believe I really went. I've been working the program for three months, haven't had a drink since day one, but he still doesn't trust me. What's wrong with him?"

There is loss of trust in *any* addiction. When someone trusts you, it means they see you as predictable and dependable, and they have faith in you. A person who is predictable will behave the same way in the future as he has in the past. A dependable person is one who can be relied on when it matters. Both predictability and dependability reflect past behavior. But since future behavior cannot always mirror the past, trust involves the belief—based on past experience that you care—that you will continue to be responsive and caring.

According to Erich Fromm, author of *The Art of Loving*, "Faith is an indispensable quality of any significant friendship or love. 'Having faith' in another person means to be certain of the reliability and unchangeability of his fundamental attitudes, of the core of his personality, of his love" (page 103). Does this description fit you? Since the time you began your involvement with chemicals, have you deserved the trust of your partner? Your children? Your employer? Your friends? Most readers of this book will admit that the answer is "no." Losing their trust took time, and so will regaining it. It will most likely take a year, not a month. The best way to rebuild trust is to be dependable and honest, day after day, one day at a time.

Here are some suggestions that will facilitate the restoration of trust in your relationship with your significant other:

- Establish your intention of being honest by disclosing, early on, all the elements of your addictive behaviors in the past, so that your partner will not have any unpleasant surprises later on. (See the section on Disclosure, in Chapter Six.)

- Be honest about the little things in your life, and your partner will eventually believe that you are likely to be honest about the big things. If you forget to run an errand that you'd promised to do, don't make up an excuse—admit you just forgot.

- Be accountable (see pp. 140-141). If you say you will be home at a certain time, be there; if you can't, telephone. If you make plans with your family, be there.

- Maintain your involvement with your recovery work. Attend twelve-step or other recovery meetings regularly, work with a sponsor, become more educated about your addiction by reading, and go to therapy. Don't just bring your body—get involved!

- Continue to disclose to your partner any lapses, slips, or relapses that are likely to have an impact on your relationship. If you are in doubt about what to disclose, talk it over with your therapist and sponsor.

# Support Groups for Family Members

Addiction is a family disease. When one member of the family is addicted, everyone else is affected. In an attempt to deal with the addict, the spouse often develops a set of beliefs and behaviors that are not helpful to the addict. For example, a wife may fear that her husband will get fired if he misses yet another day of work. When he wakes up with another hangover, she calls the boss and says her husband is ill. This behavior is called *enabling*. What it enables is for the addict to continue using without experiencing significant consequences.

Because the addict's top priority is the addiction, the spouse may feel rejected, resentful, and responsible. Some find themselves raising children virtually alone, even if they also have a full-time job. They may experience a lot of anger, which might be expressed either directly or in the form of critical remarks and put-downs. Some spouses believe that somehow they caused the addict to use, that they can somehow control the problem, and that, if only they were more perfect themselves, they could cure it. When the drinking or drugging continues despite their best efforts, they feel helpless and ineffective. They may feel shame at their inability to control the addict, and they may hide the problem from their friends and family. Some may feel very isolated and alone.

If the addict does seek help and embarks on a recovery program, some spouses may so fear another disappointment that they are unable to trust his progress. They are just waiting for the other shoe to drop, for the addict to relapse. Other spouses have gotten so used to making all the family decisions that they resist the recovering addict's attempts to get involved.

Spouses often end up as troubled as the addict. That is why they are often referred to as *co-addicts*. They have developed their own addiction-related disorder, for which they could use help. Like the addict, they can find real help by attending a mutual-support group, ideally Al-Anon, which was mentioned earlier—the twelve-step program for family and friends of alcoholics—or one of its offshoots. Progress is often quickest when the meetings are supplemented by counseling or therapy. Some of the benefits of Al-Anon are the following:

- Finding a group of people who can really understand your situation, having been there themselves.

- Recognizing you don't have to go it alone. The group, and a force greater than yourself, can help you recover.

- Learning a set of steps that can improve your self-esteem and teach you a better way of living.

- Understanding that you did not cause the problem, cannot control it, and cannot solve it.

- Changing your focus from controlling the addict to better managing your own life.

- Learning the language of recovery, so that you can better communicate with your recovering partner.

- Developing your own spirituality.

Teen-age children of alcoholics and drug addicts should attend Ala-Teen, a twelve-step program for adolescents that is based on AA but that has adult advisors.

Now that you have taken a detailed look at the damage your addiction has caused, and you have been introduced to some essential steps in recovery, it is time to begin making a new plan for your life. The next chapter will show you how.

## References

Carnes, P. *Facing the Shadow: Starting Sexual and Relationship Recovery.* (Wickenburg, Arizona: Gentle Path Press, 2001).

# CHAPTER EIGHT: A New Plan

**new** adj. *not yet familiar or accustomed*
**plan** n. *a program for making, doing, or proceeding*

Healing from addiction requires an inner determination to change what you do, minute to minute, in order to significantly alter your life. Maintaining a sustained remission requires you to balance priorities. Addicts characteristically live life with intensity and in extremes. Life is a roller-coaster ride. Mood swings, erratic hours, constantly changing goals and possibilities, new crises, and daily challenges—all combine to assure that life remains exciting and intense. Through it all, the one medication you have relied on to get you through the stress and struggles was your drug of choice. Unfortunately, this life-style is no longer working, and you are beginning to recognize this. Now is the time for a new plan.

Being aware of this is only the beginning of change. The fact is, it takes both motivation to change and skill to stay in recovery. You can be motivated, and have all the good intentions to stay sober, but, without some specific skills related to your own situation, it is unlikely you can remain in recovery. You can also have all the skills in the world, but without motivation you cannot make yourself use those skills. *It takes both motivation and skill to stay in recovery.*

# How People Change

Motivation to change is a process. Changing has to do not only with stopping your drug use, but also with *finding new solutions* to the problems the drug use created early in your drug use history.

James Prochaska, John Norcross, and Carlos DeClemente outlined this process of changing. They studied more than one thousand people who were able to stop smoking cigarettes without psychotherapy or drug rehabilitation. In their book, *Changing for Good* (1994), they outlined the six steps (or stages) that their patients encountered and passed through in order to make behavioral changes in their lives so as to end their nicotine addiction, regardless of their initial goals. Originally the researchers thought the smokers had to successfully complete each step before they could move on to the next. Early research showed that skipping steps commonly resulted in failure to complete the change process (relapse) or an incomplete change (switching drugs or only reducing use). However, subsequent research (Miller & Heather, 1998) indicated that people flow in and out of the various stages over time.

As every addict knows, a common feature of addiction is relapse. Long-term follow-up data suggest that more than 90 percent of clients will use again some time after treatment. Although this truth may sound pretty hopeless, a slip doesn't have to turn into a full-blown relapse. A common saying in Alcoholics Anonymous (AA) is *progress, not perfection.* Just as it takes a long time to become an addict, it also takes a long time to learn healthy ways to respond to the stress, anxiety, and pain of life. Relapse is just another step in the process of change that leads to stable recovery. Repeating the stages of change a number of times seems to offer a way to discover the many skills you need to continue to motivate yourself so you can maintain recovery.

Let's review the stages and see how they might apply to you:

**Stage 1:** Pre-contemplation. At this time, you really have no intention of changing. In fact, you aren't even considering that you might have a problem or that change is possible. You have experienced minimal consequences from your addiction, or you have minimized them so much in your head that you don't notice you are in hot water. Pre-comptemplators would not ordinarily pick up a book like this one unless coerced to do so. They just don't perceive they have a problem.

(Therapists and family members like to say that pre-contemplators are in denial!)

**Stage 2**: Contemplation means you are ambivalent about changing. The normal response in this stage is "yes, but. . . ." Part of you wants to change, and part wants to continue to use. During this period, you might take some actions that suggest a motivation to change, but the usual reason is to appease others or to make yourself look good. This is *first-order change*, and as we described earlier, the changes that take place will not be permanent because often a resentment grows as a result of changing only for someone else.

That is not to say that there is no merit in trying to make some change only to please someone else. In the beginning, that may be the only way you get going. But over time motivation needs to come from within you and be based on your realization that you are valuable and that you want to take care of yourself.

Contemplation usually begins when you experience frustration, fatigue, or difficulty with some specific situation in your life. You start to suffer some of the consequences of using. Eventually you become aware of your dissatisfaction and you attempt to determine what is going wrong. Perhaps suspicion of your drug use cropped up at work and someone has complained, or you missed an important deadline. Then you may become angry, depressed, or fearful that the consequences of using will bring pain and suffering to you and/or to your family. During this stage, there is much flip-flopping between rationalizing your drug use and identifying reasons for stopping. This ambivalence is normal and useful. This is the time to use the Decision-Making Matrix to help you actually see how your drug use provided some solutions in the past and how it is now causing you increasingly severe problems. This investigation helps to shift the balance over to the change side, even if the change is only to decrease your use. Using less or in different places is called *harm reduction*. If efforts to reduce the harm you might do to yourself and others are not working, you then have further evidence (and usually more consequences) that can help you decide that your best option is to completely stop your use of chemicals. As just stated, this would be a good time to revisit the Decision-Making Matrix about your own drug use.

## Exercise 1: Decision-Making Matrix

If you didn't do this exercise in Chapter Four, follow the procedure now. If you have already done the exercise, visit it again and look for what, if anything, has changed. In the upper-left-hand box, write the positive reasons for continuing to use; in the upper-right-hand box, inscribe the negative reasons for continuing to use. In the lower-left-hand box, put down the positive reasons for stopping your drug use, and in the lower-right-hand box the negative reasons for stopping. After you have completed the Decision-Making Matrix, re-examine everything you have written and try to draw some conclusions. What do you see that makes you want to move to the next stage of change?

| Positive Reasons to Use Drugs | Negative Reasons to Use Drugs |
|---|---|
|  |  |

| Positive Reasons to Stop Using Drugs | Negative Reasons to Stop Using Drugs |
|---|---|
|  |  |

**Stage 3**: Preparation describes the stage when the scale tips from ambivalence to changing. Sometimes this happens gradually, and sometimes it just fits. At this stage you actually prepare to take action. You get curious about how to make changes, what skills you need, and how to gain those skills. Although in this stage you make plans to take action, you have not yet overcome the ambivalence associated with actually implementing your plan to stop using. If you spend too little effort to learn the skills in the preparation stage, or you fail to ask for help from others and this leads to relapse, then you have returned to the precontemplation stage or have slipped or relapsed. Remember, slips and relapses, like all experiences, represent an opportunity to learn. The relapse autopsy is discussed in more detail in Chapter Eleven.

**Stage 4**: Action is the process of doing something. Choose a strategy and do it. If there is some measure of success in completing that strategy, then you keep on with the change momentum. Just as in preparation, if you stub your toe, the fear and pain may move you back into contemplation. If you do more than stub your toe, such as shoot your foot off, you usually will relapse and have to go through the previous steps again to get to taking action.

In this stage, you finally make the move for which you have been preparing. You take corrective action, which is the beginning of change. When actions are not sustained, it is easy to get discouraged and give up trying to change. Previous failed attempts at change cause you to falsely believe that you cannot stop using your drug forever. Dr. Patrick Carnes refers to long-lasting changes that originate from within your value system or your authentic self as *second-order changes*. Second-order changes are those actions that a person implements to change the dynamics of their life and life-style. Which type of change you make depends on your personal agenda. If your agenda is driven by your values, it is second-order change and is more likely to last. If your agenda is driven by fear or resentment, it is first order-change and will lead you back to relapse or cross addiction.

How do you move from action plan to actualization? You should understand some important concepts about the degree of change that is required in order to obtain your freedom from your drug addiction and to maintain a healthy, authentic recovery.

External changes that are done to appease others or to remove the pressure to change are almost always associated with secondary ulterior or unconscious motives that are not easy to identify. In many cases, you may not be able to determine whether the secondary motive was ulterior (that is, you concealed something intentionally to deceive someone) or unconscious (you never really thought about how your actions would affect someone). One type of external change is no worse than the other. They are only different aspects of internal narcissistic (self-serving) thinking and the exaggerated importance you place on your needs and desires over the needs, desires, and feelings of someone else.

Other people cannot readily determine the internal aspects of genuine change. Even highly trained addiction therapists and doctors may not recognize these features unless they are disclosed in the course of therapy. They represent a change in the way you view yourself with respect to other people and with respect to your drug of choice. This involves your emotions and your internal belief system. Self-help authors such as Stephen Covey, who wrote *The Seven Habits of Effective People,* referred to this as *radical change.* This type of change results in what the *Big Book of Alcoholics Anonymous* terms a *spiritual awakening.* It will facilitate the healing of your addiction.

Many people have been unable to believe in the prospect of healing their addiction because they have confused the terms *cure* and *healing.* Consider this quote from Shakti Gawain:

> The quality of the healing relationship rather than the technique may be the hidden foundation for healing. This special bond, created from compassion, trust, and the courage to move forward together, is what transforms the therapeutic process from curing to healing. From the joining of hearts and minds comes the realization that we are indeed one in our suffering. In the presence of this covenant, both healer and patient explore the depth of their experiences and resources. It is through this unity that both parties can indeed be healed.
>
> —Shakti Gawain

Your drug addiction is a chronic progressive disorder. It can never be cured. Some diseases and disorders can be cured, and the person suffering can be restored to a state of health and functioning comparable to that experienced prior to getting sick. For people afflicted with the life-threatening disorder of addiction, it is dangerous and unwise to consider cure. Through a program of recovery that promotes genuine change as we have described, it is possible to achieve what the mental-health-addiction clinicians now call *sustained remission*—healing.

At this time, it is only important for you to believe that healing (but not cure) of your addiction is possible. Millions of people have seen this miracle come into their lives. On pages 72 and 73 of the *Big Book* you will find the promises that you can experience in genuine recovery. They are specific aspects of the actualization of change that you can experience for yourself.

Stage 5: Maintenance. This is the hardest stage. You have to be able to deal with on-going challenges of life. Most addicts have little confidence in their ability to do this.

This stage is characterized by a period of time needed to consolidate the gains you have made by taking action. Temptations to backslide into a relapse of old behavior are often encountered even years after a change has been made. This is putting into action the material found in many relapse-prevention self-help books. Some people have large numbers of these books, as well as dozens of daily meditation books. All the right words and actions are nearby in black and white. This is a form of "recovery materialism," in which a person can become confused by the illusion of recovery without recognizing the need to live all the good words and right actions he or she professes. You need to actually put into action the changes you have already started making in your life. Use the successes you've had. Even if you are still using, you are not using drugs every minute of every day. Those times when you are not using, you are doing something right. Capitalize on those gains.

## Exercise 2: Reviewing Your Experience with Making Changes in Your Life

List five significant changes you have made in your life (up to the time when you began writing in this workbook) in attempting to control or set limits on your drug use. Many people recall changing jobs or working hours, leaving or entering into a relationship or living situation, setting spending limits, moving home, changing drugs, and so on.

1. _____
2. _____
3. _____
4. _____
5. _____

As you look at each of these, can you recall what you hoped to accomplish through this change? What did you believe would happen that led you to this course of action? Try to write down something for each of the changes you listed above.

1. _____
2. _____
3. _____
4. _____
5. _____

Can you draw any conclusions from your review of these attempts at change? Which ones worked well? Which ones less so? Note the ones that were based on external motivation (fear based, trying to please someone else) versus internal motivation (strength based, believing in and liking yourself). Which ones represent some skill deficit rather than a lack of internal motivation? Write down your thoughts on this in the lines below:

_____
_____
_____
_____
_____
_____

What is the importance of using your values to guide your behaviors? Who in your life would report on changes they see in your behavior, moods, and attitude as you implement a recovery plan? What would they notice?

_____

_____

_____

_____

_____

_____

_____

_____

_____

_____

# Basic Recovery Skills

Everyone needs four basic skills to be mentally healthy. Without mastering these skills, it is impossible to maintain sobriety. They are:

- Learn to *tolerate emotional distress* through emotional competence.

- *Control your impulses* to seek immediate avoidance of the emotional distress by learning strategies for reducing the craving or urge to use your substance and/or behavior of choice.

- *Motivate yourself* through positive self talk and catching and changing your thinking errors.

- Learn to *self-soothe in healthy ways* that honor you and those you love.

The first one is the hardest. It is connected to the other three, and it is related to being emotionally intelligent. In the past you responded to stress and anxiety by withdrawing, avoiding, or attacking yourself or others; recovery requires you to change your coping strategy. The good news is that you can learn skills that will help you.

*Tolerating emotional distress.* When you learn and activate the other three basic skills, you will be able to tolerate emotional distress. That means that you will be able to manage feeling angry, frustrated, tired, lonely, jealous, fearful, sad, as well as feeling excited, happy, and successful. Of course, you have to, first, be able to identify the emotional state and stay with it long enough to know what it is. Sometimes therapists tell you to "sit in it," meaning sit with the feeling no matter how awful it feels. That is hard if you have been spending years avoiding the feeling! However, once you are able to identify it, you can then contain it rather than swallow or stuff it down inside you. Once you are able to identify and contain the emotional state, you can then decide when and how you want to respond to it. The more you respond in ways that serve the safety, growth, and fulfillment of yourself and others, the healthier you are. You can self-regulate emotions without having to use drugs or some other avoidant or withdrawing behavior to help you get through the distress.

*Controlling impulses through delayed gratification.* If you are triggered by a situation or feeling, the trigger often can become an excuse to drink or use. The trigger initiates a chain reaction beginning with an immediate impulse to seek some way to change how you feel. If you give in to it and use, you will experience initial gratification as your unpleasant emotional state vanishes. Unfortunately, as you well know, it is a short-lived solution. But the urge to use becomes programmed into your brain as an immediate response when you get triggered. What are common situations that most addicts have when they have urges to go back to drinking or drugging? (We define urge as desire, wanting, craving, or even just thinking about a drink or a fix.) Here are a few:

- *Emotional crisis or intense stress.* This is a time when the addict in your head is hollering, "I need a drink/a fix right now!" The addict rationalizes that he or she will stop using when the crisis is over. Mismanaged anger is a key emotional state during crisis or high stress for most addicts. Learning to manage anger by identifying and dealing with the fear attached to it is the solution. Delaying drinking or using often suffices to change your mood. Call for sober support.

- *Euphoric recall.* Some addicts spend time thinking and talking about drinking or using as if it were a lost lover or best friend. They recall the feelings generated during early use, especially those that represented those first "highs." The addict frequently believes there is some way to re-create that initial feeling. Recognize that you can never regain that initial euphoria because your brain has changed. It takes more of the drug and/or added risk to re-create a similar "high." Moreover, with each using experience there are now some negative consequences.

- *Environmental triggers.* Triggers associated with the people, places, and things surrounding using can be a quick path to relapse. Knowing and avoiding them is very important. You need to learn to plan ahead for avoiding or escaping these environmental situations.

- *Testing your control.* After a period of sobriety, most addicts become overconfident and think they can manage just one drink or have drugs around without using. Even if they succeed initially, it is rare that addicts are able to resist the temptation, especially if stress and anxiety get high again—and they will, that is life. Make another choice. Distract yourself with an activity that is pleasant or that can be accomplished easily (clean out the silverware drawer or take out the trash).

- *Negative self-talk.* When something goes badly, the addict wants to get out the pity-pot and have a seat, listing for him- or herself all the negative evidence that he or she is bad, a loser, unworthy, and unlovable. This then leads to all the excuses he or she uses to use. Learning to stop the negative self-talk and doing a reliable analysis of the situation is part of what will keep you on track. Challenge your thinking errors with evidence of how you have been success-ful in this type of situation or a similar one. Repeat the healthy behavior that worked in the past to get out of this negative state.

To recap, here are some ways to manage urges to drink or use other drugs:

- Change the trigger situation: Plan ahead to avoid or leave the situation.

- Challenge your thoughts: Do you really need a drink? Is there another solution?

- Create, carry around, and refer to a card that lists the benefits of recovery on one side and the negative consequences of relapse on the other side. (See Exercise 3, Positive and Negative Consequences, below.)

- Tape to the dashboard of the car or put in your wallet near your cash and credit cards photographs of loved ones who would be disappointed if you used.

- Delay using for *15 minutes.* Urges decrease with time, especially if you are doing some self-soothing in a healthy way.

- Call someone and tell them how they can help you.

## Exercise 3:   Positive and Negative Consequences

One way to cope with thoughts about using is to consider the benefits of not using or the unpleasant things that would happen if you used again. Transfer these lists to a card you put in your wallet or purse and carry with you.

Benefits of recovery:

_____

_____

_____

_____

_____

_____

_____

_____

_____

_____

Negative consequences of using again:

_____

_____

_____

_____

_____

_____

_____

_____

_____

You have proceeded through a series of exercises designed to help you recognize the limits of your own determination, self-will, and best thinking. Now, reflect on how your strong identifications with your substances of choice create subtle but pervasive intentions. Intentions associated with using alter your state of consciousness; they subtly influence your thinking and actions even when you have not used your drug of choice for many days. Does it surprise you to hear again and again that most people who come to believe they are addicted to a substance do so only after the evidence is irrefutable? Only by looking back can you see that you had crossed a critical line separating appropriate and inappropriate use that was not visible to you until you acknowledged and truly accepted the disease concept of addiction. Once you have done so, it is easier to discover the extent to which your life, and especially your values and priorities, have drifted out of balance

# Authentic Self as Internal Motivation

We talked about first- and second-order change earlier. First-order change is superficial and done primarily to look good, but it represents a lonely, high-risk way of thinking. Second-order change, on the other hand, is the type of change we see people make when they are committed to changing because of a healthy, internal drive that says, "I am worth it. I can do this. I want to be different and everyday will do what it takes to change." One way to operate out of second-order-change thinking is to begin to rely on what we call the *authentic self*. "Authentic" is defined as trustworthy, reliable, genuine, real. When you refer back to the values-clarification work you did in Chapter Three, you will probably see those words. Most people do want to be reliable and trustworthy. They want to feel good enough about themselves to be genuine, no matter who they are with or under what circumstances. Did you include those words in your values list? Look back or complete the assignment again below.

## Exercise 4:   Values Clarification—My Authentic Self

Think about your motives and your agenda. Look back in your work for Chapter Three, Exercise 1, on values. What values did you identify there that you want to help you maintain your authentic self and move into second-order change? List those below.

_____

_____

_____

_____

_____

_____

_____

_____

_____

_____

_____

Identify the skills you need to actually use those values on a consistent basis. For example, if you listed honesty and trustworthiness, do you need to practice being honest every day? Do you need to practice disclosing to others immediately when you have lied, but you need some negotiation skills so it doesn't turn into a fight with your spouse? Do you need some listening and communicating skills so that, after owning up to a lie, you can hear and repeat back what your spouse is feeling after she or he realizes that you are still not always honest?

_____

_____

_____

_____

_____

_____

_____

_____

_____

_____

_____

Another resource you may find helpful for thinking about your authentic self and how you want to behave is a book by Don Miguel Ruiz called *The Four Agreements*. It is a short book, easy to read and understand, and the audiotape is also good. Basically, he says that if we make and keep the four agreements listed in the book, then we can get through life pretty well. See if you agree:

- Have integrity with your word. (Tell the truth, be sincere, take care of yourself by holding yourself and others accountable, don't take on other people's agendas, don't gossip. See if you can do all those things for a full day!)

- Don't take things personally. (When people do thoughtless, angry, or awful things—it is their stuff, not yours. They are doing these things because they feel insecure and/or fear something; yes, even bullies are insecure. When you don't take it personally, it removes the power of their action.)

- Don't make assumptions. (We too often make decisions or react to something in ways that hurt us and other people when we make an assumption rather than check something out first. Controlling your impulse to react long enough to really check something out, often lets you make a much better decision and renders a much better outcome.)

- Do the best you can. (When you do the best you can and remain open to learning from your successes and mistakes, rest assured that you can sleep at night.)

If you are having trouble figuring out your values, then use the four agreements for a while. See if things improve.

# Defining Your Own Sobriety

You might have heard someone say that another person is on a "dry drunk." That means they may not be drinking, but they are still acting and thinking like a drunk. Their behavior looks like someone with the *values* of an addict. In determining where you are in your recovery, it is important to recognize the differences among abstinence, sobriety, and recovery.

Let's establish some clear distinctions between abstinence and sobriety.

## Abstinence

*Abstinence can be defined as avoiding some (or all) mood-altering drugs or behaviors,* as in abstaining from alcohol or abstaining from gambling. Abstinence from all street drugs is commonly referred to as *being clean.* Traditionally, abstinence has been closely associated with avoidance of the use of alcohol in any form, yet not necessarily free from continuing an addiction to nicotine. Therefore, it is important to define the scope of abstinence. The experiences of millions of addicts who have preceded you will testify to the importance of defining specifically what classes of drugs you pledge to include in your abstinence contract, as well as any exceptions that are justified and regulated by a trusted person in your recovery network.

Abstinence is a mind-over-matter approach to drug use. Nancy Reagan emphasized this mental defense in her national campaign against drug abuse with the slogan "just say no to drugs." Many addicts have felt so much shame and hopelessness from the implication of this statement. It implies that anyone who will not abstain is weak minded or defective in some way. From this perspective, willpower is considered the primary defense against use, with the implication that those who use despite their intention to quit either cannot or will not commit themselves to abstinence. However, for most addicts, abstinence is associated with strong feelings of *determination, regret,* and *fear,* despite their will to stop using. Yet most people who are in beginning stages of recovery go through a period of abstinence where they feel these feelings and suffer through a period of craving.

*Feelings associated with abstinence* include all or most of the following:

**Determination**—having some motivation to not return to using, often fueled by fear of suffering further consequences.

**Regret**—wishing you were not an addict and that you had not suffered consequences related to a life that had become unmanageable. You wonder why you cannot control your use like many other people, and you feel self-pity.

**Resignation**—having a defeatist, depressed attitude toward your ability to make meaningful, continuing changes in your life. You may be unable to believe that the Serenity Prayer is relevant in your life. The promises of the AA *Big Book* do not seem to be coming true for you.

Common actions associated with abstinence include:

**Avoidance**—of people, places, and things associated with drug use.

**Destruction**—of any hidden supplies.

**Commitment**—to taking prescribed medications to decrease craving (for example, antidepressant medications like fluoxetine [Prozac™]) or to make drug use unrewarding (for example disulfiram [Antabuse™] or naltrexone [Revia™]).

**Agreement**—to a behavioral contract to not use again or to suffer certain consequences, such as submitting to treatment and rehabilitation in a more restrictive environment, incarceration, or significant losses in personal or professional life.

*Abstinence means staying away from drugs by mental effort.* It does not involve making any basic changes in your life or learning new skills and attitudes. Although the term *white-knuckling*, which is often applied to those who use this approach, implies that it's a real struggle, achieving abstinence was not the most painful or the most difficult part of the recovery process for most addicts.

# Sobriety

Historically, sobriety was connected with temperance and the temperance movement in the United States in the 1800s and early 1900s. Since then, sobriety has been associated with *a change in attitude toward the use of a drug or drugs of choice and a commitment to abstain from other mood-altering substances* unless required for legitimate medical problems and prescribed by a physician. It goes beyond abstinence in that one is also committed to living a drug- and alcohol-free life-style. Sobriety is also associated with the concept that one is "sober as a judge," with a clear mind and sound judgment. Sobriety is usually defined in rather black-and-white terms. You are considered to be either on the path of sobriety or on the road to slips and relapse.

Feelings associated with sobriety include some or most of the following:

**Hope**—you naturally feel hope when you can project yourself into the future and imagine a higher quality of life associated with a drug-free state of mind and body.

**Relief**—you are grateful that you no longer (or less often) feel acute conflict, pain, or cravings (episodes of intrusive drug hunger).

**Uncertainty**—you have some feelings of insecurity associated with residual guilt and shame over the "wreckage of the past," and you fear that you could relapse and experience even more consequences and pain. These feelings of uncertainty include nagging doubts about whether drug addiction is a real and incurable disease.

**Remorse**—you experience moral anguish and bitter regret for your past actions that it seems you can never fully make amends for.

Actions and experiences associated with sobriety include:

**Willingness**—recognizing that you need help and advice from other people and being willing to "go to any lengths" to establish sobriety.

**Reaching out to others**— realizing that you cannot maintain sobriety for an extended period of time alone, without the help of other people who love you and who are also committed to sobriety on the same terms as yourself.

**Commitment**—being determined to take responsibility for yourself, fulfill your promises to others, and maintain good relationships with the important people in your life. For many people, "walking the walk and not just talking the talk" is demonstrated through ongoing regular participation in a twelve-step program and meetings.

**Pride**—having a sense of accomplishment associated with escaping the tyranny of ongoing addiction to drugs.

**Conflict**—having continuing or intermittent urges to use some mood-altering substance or behavior in order to escape from the boredom, frustration (a form of anger), restlessness, or discomfort associated with sober living. If you don't see sufficient rewards from being sober, you might act out with self-defeating behaviors, such as quitting your job, leaving a committed relationship, and losing contact with your sponsor.

In addition to being powerless over the effects and timing of substance use, most people report negative life, emotional, and situational experiences that leave them feeling that their whole lives are chaotic, stressful, hectic, painful, and unpredictable. It seems like the odds are stacked against them. However, when you make decisions and take actions based on the values that represent your authentic self, you have a sense of power and hope about today. And doing things one day at a time is part of the secret to recovery.

# Recovery

Have you ever wondered why old-timers, people who haven't had a drink or snorted cocaine in ten years, still say they're "in recovery?" You may have wondered, haven't they finished recovering yet? The answer is "no." Recovery isn't an event, it's a long-term, in fact, lifetime *process*.

Recovery is learning a whole new way of living. Recovery symbolizes the addict's choice of a new life. When you believe you are worthy of a life free of drugs, you will receive the gifts of recovery.

Feelings associated with recovery include:

**Grief**. It hurts to end something that has been so familiar. It hurts to say goodbye to people who have been friends but who still use and aren't safe to be around.

**Relief**. Once you have made disclosures and you start living your life with honesty and integrity, you will find that you feel relief. No more secret life, no more having to worry about the last lie. Freedom.

**Gratitude**. When in recovery, it is common to look around and say, "Wow, I am so lucky to be here. I like my life. I like me, and I am so grateful to have my life back."

Actions associated with being in recovery include:

**Grieve.** You can do this formally by writing a letter to your drug, acknowledging how it once helped you and seemed like a reliable friend, and stating how the pain the relationship now gives you is evidence that you want another way of living and that you are saying goodbye. You will want to read this letter aloud in some formal ceremony with a sponsor, good friend, or peer from a mutual-support group like the twelve-step program. Practice setting boundaries with those people, places, and things you can no longer have in your life. Grieve those losses by acknowledging what you will miss about those people, places, and things.

Each time your partner or family member is reminded of your past behavior, he or she usually has an emotional response. It is appropriate to grieve about the pain such memories cause others. Be accountable.

**Celebrate.** For every milestone you make, it is important to feel grateful about it. You might want to make a gratitude list daily or weekly that you put on the mirror to remind yourself that some things can be celebrated every day. In the twelve-step programs, everyone celebrates when someone makes thirty days sober, ninety days, and certainly a full year or more. Take time to celebrate with those you love that you are getting through the tough times, learning, healing, and growing together.

**Slow down and have some balance.** Identify how you feel, and take time to respond to those feelings in a healthy way. Determine how much time it takes to have the important things in your life for recovery, for authentic self, and for healthy relationships. End those activities that you have done out of entitlement or sense of guilt, and engage in behaviors from a balanced, strong sense of self.

Tolerate emotional distress.

Stay in a feeling long enough to know what the feeling is. Recognize that feelings won't kill you.

**Demonstrate personal accountability on a consistent basis.** Learning from everything daily by doing Thoughts and Feelings Journals (discussed a bit later in this chapter) helps identify thinking errors and offers an opportunity to practice Step 11 of the 12 Steps of Alcoholics Anonymous. Reviewing behaviors of the day and looking at how you made matters worse *and* what you did well helps you make a plan for correcting mistakes on a regular basis.

**Improve spiritual connections.** This doesn't necessarily mean going to church or synagogue every week, although many recovering people do worship regularly. It means finding a way to connect internally with the divine spiritual force in your life. Many people do this through meditation or prayer, or by working in the garden or being out in nature.

**Maintain sobriety by continuing to do what works.** We recommend that you create a list of twelve things you can do each day that reflect your values and that help you stay sober. This list should include what you say to yourself to help remember the benefits of staying sober, as well as what activities you do—such as going to meetings and checking in with your sponsor or someone who has agreed to receive regular calls to talk about how you feel or to hear how you are being accountable. It might include daily prayer, exercise, or eating healthy 80 percent of the time. Every six months or so, you should review your list and see if something needs to be added or removed.

Recovery involves more than just learning how to stay away from your drug or behavior of choice. Saying goodbye to your addiction leaves a hole in you. It is necessary to grieve that loss and then replace it with positive, life-enhancing feelings, thoughts, and behaviors. Recovery involves doing a complete overhaul of your approach to life. It means replacing your dysfunctional core beliefs with positive, self-affirming ones. It means developing your spirituality. It means making conscious choices rather than being buffeted about. It means behaving with honesty and integrity, rather than taking the easier way to problem solving. It means that on an ongoing basis you acknowledge your mistakes, learn from them, and make amends for them. All this has to be done on a regular basis, one day at a time. In early recovery, some of the tools of twelve-step programs—such as checking in with your sponsor each day, sharing with others at meetings, and doing your own reading and writing (journaling)—can get you in the habit of living a recovery life-style. If you are thinking that this is a tall order, you are right. And when you learn to love yourself enough and see yourself as worthy, you will have the gifts of recovery.

# Growing Your Authentic Self by Creating Your Recovery Zone

## Internal versus External Motivation

We have spoken about internal motivation being driven by your authentic self and your values. Internal motivation is the strongest and best for helping you to be who you want to be in recovery.

It is also true that external motivators can help. Feelings can be external motivators. The big one is fear and her big sister—guilt; sometimes fear and guilt can help you stay out of harm's way. That's where your list of negative consequences comes in handy.

External motivators can be your family, partner, children, employer, or probation or parole officer. It can also be members of your twelve-step group, your sponsor, or what we call an "accountability partner." This is someone to whom you report about the progress and problems you are having with recovery. Sometimes partners (spouse or significant other) want to be the accountability partner. This is not recommended because it makes the relationship one of child–parent or prisoner–warden. However, if you are coming from strength in your authentic self, you will have an agreement with your partner that you will report to your partner behaviors that are not acceptable or that represent a relapse. You should want to make amends and be accountable for all relapses, so your partner can make an informed decision about his or her ability to stay in the relationship.

# Keeping Life in Balance

Patrick Carnes, a renowned expert of sex-addiction recovery, developed a useful tool many years ago that is extremely helpful in showing you when life is out of balance. It is appropriately called the Personal Craziness Index (PCI). The PCI is based on two assumptions:

1. Craziness shows itself in the day-to-day simple behaviors that represent self-maintenance.
2. Behavior signs occur in patterns.

For example, you might be focused solely on some issue of great importance, only to discover that your checking account is overdrawn because you failed to turn in billing requests and did not get paid. If this has happened, it is likely that you are also out of shirts because you haven't purchased laundry detergent nor done the laundry. If this pattern is pervasive, family members are complaining, you are avoiding or defending yourself, and your life feels emotionally overdrawn as well.

Addicts are famous for neglecting the basics in life. The PCI serves as a reminder each day of what we need to do.

## Exercise 5:   Personal Craziness Index (PCI)

The process of creating your own PCI is designed to be as value-free as possible. You will generate the behavioral signs (we call them *critical incidents*) that through your own experience you have learned are warning signals that you are getting out of balance, losing it, or about to crash. Therefore, it will be by your own standards that you prepare the danger signs. Dr. Carnes suggested twelve areas of personal behavior, but you may substitute or add your own as well.

**1. Physical Health**—The ultimate insanity is not to take care of our bodies. Without our bodies we have nothing, yet we seem to have little time for physical conditioning. Examples are being over a certain weight, having missed regular exercise for two days, smoking more cigarettes than normal, being exhausted from lack of sleep. How do you know that you are not taking care of your body? (at least three examples)

_____

_____

_____

_____

**2. Transportation**—How people get from place to place is often a statement about their lifestyles. Take, for example, a car owner who seldom comes to a full stop, routinely exceeds the speed limit, runs out of gas, does not check the oil, puts off needed repairs, has not cleaned the back seat in three months, and averages three speeding tickets and ten parking tickets a year. Or the bus rider who always misses the bus, never has change, forgets his or her briefcase on the bus, etc. What are the transportation behaviors that indicate your life is getting out of control? (at least three examples)

_____

_____

_____

_____

**3. Environment**—To not have time to do our personal chores is a comment on the order of your life. Consider the home in which plants go unwatered, fish unfed, grocery supplies depleted, laundry not done or put away, cleaning neglected, dishes unwashed, etc. What are ways in which you neglect your home or living space? (at least three examples)

_____

_____

_____

_____

**4. Work**—Chaos at work is risky for recovery. Signs of chaotic behavior are phone calls not returned in twenty-four hours, chronic lateness for appointments, being behind in promised work, an unmanageable in-basket, and "too many irons in the fire." When your life is unmanageable at work, what are your behaviors? (at least three examples)

_____

_____

_____

_____

**5. Interests**—What are some positive interests besides work that give you perspective on the world? Music, reading, photography, fishing, or gardening are examples. What interests do you neglect when you are overextended? (at least three examples)

_____

_____

_____

_____

**6. Social Life**—Think of friends in your social network who constitute significant support for you and are not family or significant others. When you become isolated, alienated, or disconnected, what behaviors are typical of you? (at least three examples)

_____

_____

_____

_____

**7. Family/Significant Others**—When you are disconnected from those closest to you, what is your behavior like? Examples are silent, overtly hostile, passive-aggressive. (at least three examples)

_____

_____

_____

_____

**8. Finances**—We handle our financial resources much like our personal ones. Thus, when your checking account is unbalanced, or worse, overdrawn, or bills are overdue, or there is no cash in your pocket, or you are spending more than you earn, your financial overextension may parallel your emotional bankruptcy. List the signs that show when you are financially overextended. (at least three examples)

_____

_____

_____

_____

**9. Spiritual Life and Personal Reflection**—Spirituality can be diverse and include such methods as meditation, yoga, and prayer. Personal reflection includes keeping a personal journal, completing daily readings, and pursuing therapy. What are sources of routine personal reflection that are neglected when you are overextended? (at least three examples)

_____

_____

_____

_____

**10. Other Addictions or Symptom Behaviors**—Compulsive behaviors that have negative consequences are symptomatic of your general well-being or the state of your overall recovery. When you watch inordinate amounts of TV, overeat, bite your nails–any habit you feel bad about afterward–these can be signs of burnout or possible relapse. Symptom behaviors that are evidence of overextension are those such as forgetfulness, slips of the tongue, or jealousy. What negative addiction or symptom behaviors are present when you are "on the edge?" (at least three examples)

_____

_____

_____

_____

**11. Twelve Step Practice**—Living a Twelve Step way of life involves many practices. When done consistently, they can be key to staying in your recovery zone. Group attendance, Step work, sponsorship, service, and Twelve Step calls become the foundation of a good recovery. Which recovery activities do you neglect first when you are leaving your recovery zone? (at least three examples)

_____

_____

_____

_____

**12. Sexuality**—For sex addicts, monitoring yourself sexually becomes very important. You must notice if there are sexual signs that you are not doing well, such as cravings for old behaviors, feelings of shame around sexual issues, or sexual aversion toward your partner. Also, there are the things you may be working on to improve your sexual life. What do you notice that happens (or doesn't happen) sexually that tells you things are not going well? (at least three examples)

_____

_____

_____

_____

# Recording Your PCI

The PCI is effective only when a careful record is maintained. Recording your daily progress in conjunction with regular journal-keeping will help you to stay focused on priorities that keep life manageable; work on program efforts a day at a time; expand your knowledge of personal patterns; provide a warning in periods of vulnerability to self-destructive cycles or addictive relapse.

From thirty-six or more signs of personal craziness you recorded, choose the seven that are the most critical for you. At the end of each day, review the list of seven key signs and count the ones you did that day, giving each behavior one point. Record your total for that day in the space provided on the chart. If you fail to record the number of points each day, that day receives an automatic score of seven. If you cannot even do your score, you are obviously out of balance. At the end of the week, total your seven daily scores and make an "X" on the graph. Pause and reflect on where you are in the recovery. Chart your progress over a twelve-week period.

*My seven key signs of personal craziness:*

1. _____
2. _____
3. _____
4. _____
5. _____
6. _____
7. _____

## Personal Craziness Worksheet

| DAY/WEEK | 1 | 2 | 3 | 4 | 5 | 6 | 7 | 8 | 9 | 10 | 11 | 12 |
|---|---|---|---|---|---|---|---|---|---|---|---|---|
| Sunday | | | | | | | | | | | | |
| Monday | | | | | | | | | | | | |
| Tuesday | | | | | | | | | | | | |
| Wednesday | | | | | | | | | | | | |
| Thursday | | | | | | | | | | | | |
| Friday | | | | | | | | | | | | |
| Saturday | | | | | | | | | | | | |
| Weekly Total | | | | | | | | | | | | |

# Interpretation and Use of the PCI

The PCI is useful in early recovery as recovery habits are established. Also, the PCI becomes helpful during periods of stress and vulnerability. Many simply use it as a daily reminder of their progress. These users change the items as they progress in their recovery.

## PCI Graph

| | | | | | | | | | | | | | |
|---|---|---|---|---|---|---|---|---|---|---|---|---|---|
| 50 — VERY HIGH RISK | | | | | | | | | | | | | |
| 40 — HIGH RISK | | | | | | | | | | | | | |
| 30 — MEDIUM RISK | | | | | | | | | | | | | |
| 20 — STABLE SOLIDITY | | | | | | | | | | | | | |
| 10 — OPTIMUM HEALTH | | | | | | | | | | | | | |
| 0 — | | | | | | | | | | | | | |

To use the PCI, select seven items from the "critical incidents" you have already listed. Then following the worksheet instructions, you can generate a weekly score ranging from 0 to 49. A guideline for understanding your score follows.

| OPTIMUM HEALTH 0-9 | Very resilient. Knows limits; has clear priorities; congruent with values; rooted in diversity; supportive; has established a personal system; balanced, orderly, resolves crises quickly; capacity to sustain spontaneity; shows creative discipline. |
|---|---|
| STABLE SOLIDITY 10-19 | Resilient. Recognizes human limits; does not pretend to be more than he or she is; maintains most boundaries; well ordered; typically feels competent, feels supported, able to weather crisis. |
| MEDIUM RISK 20-29 | Vulnerable to relapse. Slipping; often rushed; can't get it all in; no emotional margin for crisis; vulnerable to slip into old patterns; typically lives as if he or she has inordinate influence over others and/or feels inadequate. |
| HIGH RISK 30-39 | Relapse potential. Living in extremes (overactive or inactive); relationships abbreviated; feels irresponsible and is; constantly has reasons for not following through; lives one way, talks another; works hard to catch up. |
| VERY HIGH RISK 40-49 | Relapse probable. Usually pursuing self-destructive behavior; often totally in mission or cause or project; blames others for failures; seldom produces on time; controversial in community; success vs. achievement-oriented. |

# Seeking Professional Help

You may be well into the process of recovery but find that you are triggered to use and just can't get beyond memories of past traumas or anger and resentment of past and current problems. Perhaps you have another condition that makes recovery more difficult, such as bipolar illness or depression. It is important to seek professional help for these conditions. Using the skills of a therapist and/or psychiatrist can be the additional support you need to really be able to get into a recovery zone.

# Taking Time to Think through Journaling

Have you ever heard of Antabuse™ (disulfiram), a drug that is used to help alcoholics remain abstinent? It works by stopping the breakdown of alcohol in the liver part way through the process, leading to the accumulation of a toxic breakdown product in the body. This chemical is not dangerous, but it causes the person to feel very, very ill. The obvious way to prevent this misery is to avoid drinking any alcoholic beverage. Most slips occur because the person has impulsively taken a drink, telling himself, "it's just one—I can handle it," or, "I've had such a bad day—I've got to have this," or, "I've done so well that I deserve to reward myself." What (disulfiram) Antabuse™ does is make a person *think*. If you have (disulfiram) Antabuse™ on board, the minute you are tempted, a little voice inside you will say, "but if I take this drink, I will pay for it in a big way!" So you decide to take a pass on the drink.

Addicts tend to live in the moment. Once you have, apparently on impulse, taken the first step on the path to using again, it becomes progressively harder to stop yourself from using. It is paradoxical that, although most addicts who are still drinking and using believe they can control their drinking, they also believe that in many ways life controls *them*. When you say, "I drank because my boss chewed me out," or "I used because I happened to drive by my dealer's house," or "I took a hit because my friend offered it to me," you are demonstrating a belief that you have no choices, that you are a victim of circumstances and of other people. You are saying that when someone else yells, "jump!" you instinctively ask, "how high?" as you prepare to jump.

In recovery, it is important to learn to live consciously. This means that you recognize you have choices instead of reacting automatically. Before you act, learn to monitor what you are saying to yourself about what happened and to access the feelings behind those thoughts. You can then ask yourself, does my first reaction make sense? Are there other possible reactions in this situation? What are my options for how to respond? Would snorting some coke be my best reaction? What are the consequences for me? This process is hard for most people, but it is especially hard for addicts, most of whom learned long ago to suppress and discount their feelings and not think through their actions.

Journaling about your thoughts and feelings is a great way to develop the skills you need for conscious living. The exercises that you have been doing in this workbook have already given you practice in writing down things about yourself. You may wonder, what should I write down? Here are some suggestions:

- If something good unexpectedly happened to you today, write what happened and how you felt about it, and thank your higher power for continuing to watch out for you. Develop a mindset to notice all those little things that work out for you each day, and write them down, along with your feelings of gratitude. The twelve-step program encourages an "attitude of gratitude," and this requires conscious attention.

- If you were tempted to drink or use today but didn't, describe what happened. If the drink or drug was actually there, write down how you happened to be in a place where the opportunity was present and how you met the challenge. If you were elsewhere when the desire or urge came into your head, try to reconstruct what happened in your life just before you thought of using that might have led to the desire. Then write down the sequence of things you said to yourself and the actions you took that helped you decide not to take action to use. Write down your feelings about having been able to make this decision.

- If you did use, write down a narrative similar to the one above. Record your thoughts and feelings that led you to use, and how you felt about it afterwards. Think about what you might do or say to yourself differently next time so that the outcome is better, and how you imagine you would feel about it.

- If you handled some situation well today, write it down. For example, if your spouse had a complaint and you listened quietly instead of becoming defensive and arguing, write what happened and how you were able to respond differently from your usual pattern. Record how you feel about the way you responded.

- If something got you upset today, write what happened, what your thoughts and feelings were at the time, how you feel about it now, and how you would ideally handle this situation.

## Exercise 6:   Thoughts and Feelings Journals

Below is one model you might use for recording the events in your life. You will find a journal on page 273 that is easy to copy so you can use a new one each time you want to write about a different event or situation. You will be pleasantly surprised at how quickly daily use of such a journal can help you understand yourself and change your actions, thoughts, and feelings.

**Thoughts–Feelings Journal**                    **Date_____**

**Event or situation**

_____

_____

_____

**What happened?**

_____

_____

_____

**Who was there?**

_____

_____

_____

## When and where?

_____

_____

_____

## Thoughts

What thoughts were going through your head just before the event, during the event, and immediately after the event? Circle the thoughts that may be related to your core beliefs about yourself.

_____

_____

_____

_____

_____

_____

_____

_____

_____

_____

## Emotions

What emotions did you feel? Underline the strongest two feelings. Circle feelings that are triggers for you to want to act out.

_____

_____

_____

## Body sensations

Often the body gives us a signal that something is going on before we are really aware that we may be in a bad place. Listen to your body. Describe any body sensations you felt during the process.

_____

_____

_____

What does your body do when you get angry or sad?

_____

_____

_____

How does it tell you that you are having a strong feeling or reaction?

_____

_____

_____

## What I did well

_____

_____

_____

When we've gotten into a highly emotional situation that we've mismanaged, we think we made a mess of everything. This section is to remind you that you did do something right (usually). Think about what part of the situation you handled well or did not make worse. Note those items here.

_____

_____

_____

## How I made things worse

In this section, list the ways you made the situation worse.

_____

_____

_____

## Thinking errors

Look at your thoughts from section 2 (Thoughts) of this journal entry. Are any of those thoughts thinking errors? Actively search for information or evidence that contradicts the thoughts or that supports the thoughts.

_____

_____

_____

_____

_____

_____

_____

_____

_____

_____

Over the past few years, Tiger Woods has risen from the ranks of professional golfers to become recognized as a master in the sport. He refers to his mental attitude toward the game as "being in the zone."

## Exercise 7:   Getting into a Zone

In this exercise you will practice learning to focus on what will help you maintain your recovery.

First, sit with both feet touching the floor and with a straight spine so that you are able to feel the air going in and out of your lungs, forcing your diaphragm up and down. Focus on your breathing. With each out-breath, breathe out all the feelings you do not need (fear, anger, resentment, self-doubt.) With each in-breath, let in all the feelings you need (serenity, strength, love, confidence, humility). Do this through six breaths, or until you firmly know the feeling states that hold you back and the feeling states that you think reflect those of a strong person in recovery.

Now think of a time when you were younger, when you felt strong and enthusiastic about life. Perhaps a time when you were resting in a special place where you could daydream and experience a sense of wonder at the world that surrounds you. A time when you believed that all things were possible. A time when you believed that, if you placed all of your heart, spirit, and energy into a goal, you could accomplish anything. A time when all possibilities were within reach, when your emotions were attuned and balanced, and you felt physically capable of doing anything. Consider how old you were at this time.

Now think of times as an adult when you felt you were close to optimal performance. What were you doing? Where were you? Was anyone else present? What were you thinking about yourself? What else were you doing in your life that was productive? List that information below.

_____

_____

_____

_____

_____

_____

_____

_____

_____

_____

Now, reflect upon these peak interludes in your life for a minute. Can you identify a few common feelings or qualities or characteristics you associate with them? List them below.

_____

_____

_____

_____

_____

_____

_____

_____

_____

_____

Now, close your eyes and visualize yourself as having these feelings, qualities, or characteristics today. Do this every day for two weeks, and then determine if this activity should be on your daily activities list.

If you find that you don't remember any times where you were successful, think of someone whom you think is consistently authentic. It may be a spiritual leader whom you want to study or already know something about. List the qualities this person has and then daily visualize yourself as having at least one of the qualities.

Being able to identify these features is of great benefit as you try to determine the spaces and places in your day-to-day life that give you optimum physical, mental, spiritual, and psychological health. We call this sense of well-being the *recovery zone.*

Through the practice of positive imagery each day, like Tiger Woods you are setting up the optimal conditions for your brain to remember and to help you take actions from a place of strength and confidence rather than fear.

Recovery requires lots of work on your part, and most people recognize it is impossible to do this all by yourself. The next chapter tells you how to create your recovery support community. These are the people who can help you learn the skills for recovery, be accountable, and celebrate your recovery.

## References

Alcoholics Anonymous World Services (1972 ). *Alcoholics Anonymous, 3rd Edition.* New York: Author.

Covey, S. (1989) *The Seven Habits of Effective People.* New York: Simon & Schuster.

Gawain, S. (1978) *Creative Visualization.* New York: Bantam Books.

Miller, W. & Heather, N. Eds. (1998) *Treating Addictive Behaviors. 2nd Edition.* New York: Plenum Press.

Prochaska, J.O, Norcross, J.C., and DiClemente, C.C. (1994). *Changing for Good* New York, NY: William Morrow and Co.

Ruiz, Don Miguel(1999) *The Four Agreements.* New York: Simon and Schuster.

# CHAPTER NINE: Creating Your Recovery Support Community

**create** v. *to bring about*
**support** v. *to help, comfort, bring courage, faith or confidence to*

It is difficult to recover alone. Experience has shown that you must first join with others and form an alliance in order to unconditionally surrender to a process that can lead from drug addiction to freedom. The disease of addiction is too powerful for any one of us to overcome it by ourselves. By joining with others who also seek the goals of healing and freedom, you may yet succeed! Your capacity to join with others in this common cause has been shown by your determination to keep working through this book. You could not have fully and effectively completed the exercises in the previous chapters without assistance from others.

# Developing Twelve-Step Support

Just as there are many ways to worship God, there are many ways to recover from addictions. This book emphasizes the Twelve-Step program of Alcoholics Anonymous (AA) because it is an effective, well-known path to recovery, and it is the path taken by most addicts who seek help from others. Later in this chapter we will describe some other ways to recovery. All have some basic principles in common. For now, we will continue with guidelines for twelve-step recovery. One of its major elements is getting support from others. Here are some suggestions for getting the most benefit from your twelve-step support system:

1. **Learn from people with significant recovery**.

   Sharing faith, hope, and experience is a vital part of every recovering person's life. This is one of the most rewarding activities you can do. As you find others to teach you about what has helped and hurt their recovery, you will develop new perspectives and skills.

2. **Learn to communicate with others.**

   Overcoming the fear of reaching out to others when you are craving or tempted to use is critical if you want to remain free from your addiction. Even though it may be difficult, use the phone to call group members and sponsors as many times as necessary. Create a *call list*, which is a list of people who agree to be called at any time to help you through a tough time. (Sometimes people do agree to be on your call list, but they establish limits to times when they can be available. This is a good boundary to set for folks with children or other responsibilities. It doesn't mean that that person won't be there for you; it just means that you have to plan for times when you will call another person on the list.)

   It is also important to figure out what helps you when you are triggered, so you can tell people on your call list what you need. That way, when you make the call, they can provide meaningful support. For example, if all you need is for someone to listen to how hard things are right now, rather than create a solution for you, it is important to tell those on your call list—when you call—that all you need is a listener. If you need someone to tell you to get to a meeting or to come pick you up for a meeting, communicate that to the person. If you need them to ask you what would be a solution, so you are forced to think through one, request that. You get the idea—you have to *communicate* what you need when you reach out.

3. **Be patient.**

   There are no short cuts or magical incantations that will bring you to a speedy cure. Daily application of the program principles and growth along spiritual lines is the only path to genuine, lasting recovery.

4. **Go to meetings consistently.**

   You will find groups promoting healthy recovery if you continue to search. Or help create one that will meet your needs. This is your lifeline, your support network—so be proactive. If the meeting does not fit your needs after a couple of tries, then try another. Meetings, like people, vary, so try several until you find your fit.

5. **Use your sponsor(s).**

   A sponsor is someone who uses the twelve-step program in his or her daily life and is willing to be in a relationship with you that is nonsexual and nonexploitative for the purpose of helping you apply the program to your life. You can always ask for a temporary sponsor until you get to know him and he gets to know you. This way, if it isn't working out for either of you, you can get another temporary sponsor until you find a good match—someone who listens and shares or gives desired direction if you are stuck.

6. **Use program literature.**

   Program-approved reading material is available at meetings and through sponsors. You can obtain it through phone calls and Internet resources. The material is of value only if you use it. People report that completing the step work of the traditional Twelve Steps is very helpful to provide a process for thinking through your situation and creating solutions.

7. **Maintain contact outside the meetings.**

   The meetings represent the recovery community in session. In addition to the meetings, group members create other activities to promote recovery and celebrate living life each day. It is a good way to practice social skills, too. If you found in past social situations that you felt comfortable only when you were using, then finding ways to share in outside activities with other recovering people will allow you to practice having fun without pressure to use.

# Knowing the Signs of a Healthy Twelve-Step Group

When Reggie had a physical exam, his doctor noticed a hole in the membrane between his nostrils. That's when Reggie admitted he was addicted to snorting cocaine and in fact he was having financial problems because of it. The doctor strongly recommended that Reggie attend a meeting of Narcotics Anonymous, and that evening Reggie went to his first meeting. In the room he found ten other people, all of them relative newcomers except for one person with more than a year's sobriety. It was a discussion meeting, and most of the sharings were detailed descriptions of urges and cravings and how they had led to relapses. No one offered any solutions, and by the time Reggie left he had a strong desire to use and felt discouraged about any likelihood of recovery. He headed straight for his dealer's house, telling himself, "I'm never going back to an NA meeting again!"

Not all twelve-step meetings are the same. If you look inside your local AA meeting guide, you will see that there are several types of meetings, which differ in their format:

- At speakers' meetings, one or more people tell the story of their addiction and their recovery, while the rest of the group listens and learns.

- At discussion meetings, everyone takes turns briefly sharing their recent experiences, feelings, and problems. Sometimes the sharing is about some specific topic that was announced at the beginning of the meeting. Others do not interrupt or ask questions, but subsequent speakers often respond by relating how they had similar feelings, or how they solved the problem or dealt with the topic.

- At step meetings, one of the Twelve Steps or traditions is read, and the ensuing shared information is focused on how that particular step was played out in the speaker's life.

- "Closed" meetings are open only to people with the addiction on which that particular twelve-step group focuses, whereas "open" meetings are open to everyone. Family members and friends who are interested in learning more are welcome at "open" meetings.

Meetings also differ in the type of audience they are meant for. In cities where there are many meetings, some may be specifically for:

- Newcomers

- Old-timers or more seasoned members

- Women

- Gays, lesbians, and transgendered persons

- Nonsmokers

Finally, meetings differ in how healthy they are. This depends on who attends, how they behave, how they adhere to the twelve traditions (which are guidelines for twelve-step groups) and whether they are focused on "the problem" or on solutions. Here are some guidelines for what constitutes a healthy twelve-step meeting:

- The people are there to learn the tools of recovery, not just to socialize.

- The meeting needs to feel like a safe place, so maintaining the rules of confidentiality and anonymity is crucial. "What is said here, stays here" is the general rule. Members do not gossip to outsiders about what was said at the meeting. Members do not use the meeting to find sexual partners, "using" friends, or customers for their business.

- The traditional guidelines of twelve-step meetings are followed— no interrupting, no advice giving, no self-promotion.

- The people there include those with experience in a twelve-step program, who can keep the meeting on track. For example, recognizing that newcomers are easily triggered to act out, the more seasoned members can point out that one person's detailed descriptions of his or her addictive behavior can trigger others; it is better for the speaker to mention briefly what happened and then focus on one's feelings and attempts to solve the problem.

- The focus of the meeting is on applying the principles of the program in people's lives, not on sharing their misery or their acting out.

- Newcomers are encouraged to obtain a temporary sponsor (a discussion about sponsors follows), and veteran members are encouraged to take on this responsibility.

- Leadership of the meeting is shared—there is no one "guru" who dominates the group.

## Exercise 1:  Observing

At your next twelve-step meeting, notice how well the meeting follows the previously mentioned guidelines. If the answer is "poorly," then you may be better off attending a different meeting.

# Developing and Maintaining a Relationship with a Sponsor

This book has already mentioned sponsors more than once. A sponsor is a person with more experience in the program who helps you work the Twelve Steps. The sponsor explains the basic concepts and language of the program, answers your questions, confronts your behavior when necessary, is available during your difficult times, gives you practice in building relationships, and, most important, models the twelve step program in his or her own life. A good resource for understanding the roles and responsibilities of sponsors and sponsees is *Twelve Step Sponsorship: How it Works* by Hamilton B. On page 3, Hamilton lists the following major elements of the sponsor-sponsee relationship:

- The primary responsibility of sponsors is to help their sponsees work the Twelve Steps.

- A sponsor and a sponsee have an obligation to discuss their mutual expectations, objectives, and requirements, if any, regarding the sponsorship relationship *before* they enter into that relationship.

- A sponsor shares his or her experience, strength, and hope with the sponsee, rather than trying to run the sponsee's life.

- A sponsor must never take advantage of a sponsee in any way.

A newcomer to the twelve-step program is a very vulnerable person, and the sponsor-sponsee relationship is one of trust and intimacy. To minimize the risk of a romantic or sexual relationship between sponsor and sponsee, it is recommended that heterosexual newcomers choose a member of the same sex as a sponsor. If a gay recovering person is considering sponsoring a same-sex newcomer, don't agree to sponsor that newcomer if you believe that either of you might have a romantic interest in the other; if such feelings do develop, break off the sponsorship.

In choosing a sponsor, look for someone at meetings whom you respect and want to emulate. He or she needs to have more time than you in twelve-step recovery, to be living his life according to the Twelve Steps, and to be practicing the spiritual aspects of the program. He needs to have the time to be available to you on a regular basis as well as at any time for emergencies. Remember that such people are often much in demand as sponsors, so if you approach this person and are turned down, don't take it personally—look for someone else with similar qualifications.

# Managing Conflicts between One's Relationship and Recovery Activities

For years, Mario had a well-established pattern of calming himself after a stressful day at the office. He had a standing date to meet some buddies at the bar on the way home. There, they would shoot the breeze, down a few beers, and unwind. By the time he'd get home, he'd be much more relaxed and more ready to face Marissa and her various demands. Unfortunately, much of the time it was quite late by the time he got home. He knew this made her unhappy, but he also knew he'd be a bear if he went directly home at the end of the day. When he got his second DUI after leaving the bar, Mario realized it was time for a change.

Marissa was thrilled when Mario stopped drinking. Although he was mandated by the court to attend the meetings, he liked them and he seemed sincere in his desire to stay sober. But when he came home and told her that his new sponsor had suggested he go to ninety meetings in ninety days, most of them in the evening, Marissa hit the roof:

"Before, you were out every evening drinking. Now you're out every evening at some meeting. I don't see that anything has changed!! Isn't it about time you started spending the evening with me and the kids?"

If you have found yourself in this common situation, you probably felt caught in the middle. You may feel guilty about continuing to leave your spouse alone at home, but at the same time you know that the best thing for your recovery right now is to attend those meetings. What can you do?

The first thing you need to realize is that without personal recovery, you will never be the spouse your partner wants you to be. In the early weeks and months, your own recovery has to come first—ahead of your marriage, your job, and everything else. The time you spend right now in recovery work is an investment in your—and your relationship's—future. Your goal is to help your spouse see this, so that she will support you in your twelve-step involvement.

One way to do this is to help your spouse understand that addiction is a family disease. Everyone in your family has been affected by your addiction. It is entirely understandable that by now your spouse is resentful of your absences, angry with you, upset at herself for her inability to control your drinking, and distrustful of your actions. One thing you can do to help is to ask her (or him) how she or he is feeling and what you can do at this moment that might help. Then make an attempt to do what is requested. If it is impossible, offer an alternative. Most important, reassure your partner that you love her or him. The best thing your partner can do to combat the feeling of being less important to you than your meetings is to get some education about addiction and her own reactions. A good way she can do this is to attend Al-Anon or equivalent, a twelve-step program for families and friends of alcoholics and drug addicts. If your partner says, "I don't need a meeting—*I'm* not the one with the problem!" ask her or him to go for your sake. For example, by becoming familiar with twelve-step language and principles, the two of you will be able to communicate more effectively with each other about your recovery. Many family members of addicts began attending Al-Anon meetings in order to help the addict—and continued to go because they realized it was helping themselves. The couple relationship usually does better when *both* members of the couple are attending twelve-step meetings.

If you go back to the end of Chapter Seven you will see a list of the benefits for family members who attend Al-Anon and related meetings. Review this list and show it to your partner. If you are involved in an outpatient drug-addiction program, it is likely that the program will encourage your spouse to attend its sessions as well as Al-Anon.

You should also check out whether your city has meetings of Recovering Couples Anonymous (RCA), a twelve-step program for couples recovering from *any* addiction. These meetings usually focus on some aspect of recovery that is rarely discussed in the separate AA and Al-Anon meetings. For example, one week the subject may be "balancing individual and couple needs." The following week the focus may be "rebuilding trust," or "forgiveness," or "improving our sex life," or "handling our finances." As a newcomer to these meetings, you and your partner will learn firsthand how other couples have handled these issues. The meetings are usually held monthly. The only difference in format between these meetings and other twelve-step meetings is that after one member of the couple shares, the other member of the couple has the first opportunity to speak next. These meetings are definitely *not* a forum for complaining about your partner, but rather for presenting problems and solutions. No one is obligated to say anything. You can find contact information for RCA in Appendix B.

After your first ninety days, it is time to think about making some compromises. At this point you may find that three or four meetings a week are sufficient for you. Plan on spending some quality time with your partner—for example, you might agree to a weekly date together, without the kids, so that you can get to know each other again. Many alcoholics have never had sex while sober, so this is a time to renew your sexual relationship with your partner. And here's another tip—during your drinking and using days, your addiction had top priority, and your partner was well aware of this. He or she most likely felt neglected. If you now demonstrate to your partner that you think about her, love her, and are behaving more responsibly toward her, she will be more comfortable with your need to leave the house for meetings.

Phone your partner at some point during the day and say "I've been thinking about you and I'm grateful you're sticking by me," or something of the sort. (Of course, this will be effective only if you are sincere, not if you do it out of obligation!)

Notice the ways in which you may have been putting down, discounting, and dismissing your partner's concerns, requests, and complaints (this is actually part of your Tenth Step work), and see how often you can stop yourself before the words leave your mouth. Instead, first listen seriously to what your partner is telling you, and then respond respectfully. You and your partner may need the coaching of a couples' counselor if this turns out to be too difficult a task.

# Engaging in Service Activities with Others

In the old days, many psychiatrists believed that there was such a thing as an "addictive personality." Because addicts are often so self-centered and put their own needs ahead of everyone else's, they were thought to have a "narcissistic" or "antisocial" personality disorder. Some addicts certainly do, just as some nonaddicts have personality disorders. The amazing fact, however, is that for most addicts these apparent personality disorders diminish as they begin to live a sober life. It is now understood that self-centeredness is part of addictive disorders.

Unfortunately, after focusing on their addiction for so many years, recovering addicts are often rusty in their service skills. One of the many benefits of twelve-step programs is that they give people practice in these skills so that they become more comfortable carrying them out in various aspects of their life. Agreeing to service activities also means you are committing to being responsible and following through, which are additional skills that many addicts need to learn.

When you join a twelve-step group, you will be given opportunities to be of service to others. These activities are not obligatory (nothing is obligatory in AA; even the Twelve Steps themselves are "suggested" rather than required), but we recommend that you take advantage of these opportunities. Some of these are:

- Driving someone to a meeting or back home afterwards

- Arriving early to open up the meeting room and arrange the chairs

- Rearranging the chairs after the meeting ends and locking up the meeting room

- Bringing twelve-step literature with you to the meetings

- Making coffee at the meeting

- Talking after the meeting with someone who seems to need help.

After some period of sobriety, you will have additional opportunities for service, such as:

- Being a sponsor

- Going with another member of the group to make a "twelfth-step call" on an addict who has asked for help

- Taking a turn chairing the meeting

- Joining a committee of your fellowship, such as a prison outreach committee, literature committee, and so forth

# Identifying a Sobriety Celebration Date

For many recovering addicts, a sobriety birthday is more important than the anniversary of your birth. Getting to one year of sobriety is a major accomplishment! So is celebrating the first six months of sobriety, the first three months, and, for a newcomer, the first month without drinking and drugging. It is validating to get recognition for these accomplishments. You probably remember exactly when you had your last drink or last cocaine binge, so it isn't difficult to calculate how long it's been since then. You deserve to celebrate! Twelve-step groups have chips for various milestones of sobriety. Let yourself be congratulated on these occasions. When you make it to one year, make it a big occasion within your recovery meetings! (Try to be sensitive that not all partners are thrilled to be reminded of all the pain that has come with the addiction when the sobriety date rolls around. It is helpful to talk with your spouse or partner before the date to determine what you, as a couple, have to celebrate from the past year. Some couples talk about the positive and negative impact of the addiction prior to the anniversary date of sobriety. Giving your partner the choice to be part of the celebration, or not, is a way to be respectful of the mixed feelings that happen for most partners.)

When thinking about how to celebrate sobriety dates, here are some considerations. First, like most addicts, you probably are an expert at justifying drinking or using. You've probably said to yourself in the past, "I've worked so hard and am so hot and tired, I deserve a drink." Or, "I just got this promotion—it's time to party." *Don't* use the occasion of a sobriety birthday to drink or use! Although it sounds crazy to do so, don't be surprised if the thought enters your head or if you think you can challenge yourself to just one drink or snort—one is a relapse and it invites your brain to feel wounded again and ask for more.

Second, if you are being treated by a physician for a medical or psychiatric disorder with various drugs, you might wonder whether you are indeed "sober" and entitled to celebrate a sobriety date. AA clearly states that medications that are prescribed by a physician and that are being used as prescribed *do not* constitute a break in sobriety [AA World Services, 1994]. This includes anti-depressants, anti-anxiety drugs, and even opioids (narcotics) prescribed for chronic pain. If your sponsor or other individuals in your twelve-step program do not agree with this principle, find a different sponsor.

Finally, remember that relapses are a well-known part of addictive disorders. Did you know that the average heavy cigarette smoker has quit more than four times before he or she succeeds in quitting permanently? Many alcoholics and addicts relapse, especially in their first few months of sobriety. Unfortunately, a relapse is also a time for shame. Alcoholics and other addicts already have a lot to be ashamed about, and setting back your sobriety date is usually another. Just remember that many long-timers in AA, the folks who are celebrating their tenth or twentieth or thirtieth AA birthday, had to set their sobriety date back more than once before they got to those birthdays. A relapse is a learning opportunity. It is a time to strengthen your program and to review the steps that led to the relapse so you can prevent the next one.

# Alternative Support for Getting Sober

By now it must be clear to you that recovery from addiction is most efficiently approached with a combination of formal treatment and group support. These are two different modalities, although they may overlap. *Treatment* implies paying a trained professional to work with you, which may be in an individual or a group setting. The professional supports you, listens to you, confronts you over your errors in judgment or unhelpful behavior, makes suggestions, gives homework assignments, and educates you. The professional may or may not be a recovering addict, but he or she has expertise in treating addiction. The relationship between you and the professional is not a peer relationship.

*Self-help* or *mutual support group* implies a group of people, most often addicted to the same drug or behavior, who get together to support each other in their recovery. Although some have had more time and more success than others, they are basically peers (equals). Some self-help groups are led by professionals, whereas others are not. In these latter groups, there is usually a tradition that someone with experience in the group's program leads. By far the most common self-help program in the United States and other countries is Alcoholics Anonymous and its offshoots. That's why this book devotes a lot of space to AA's Twelve Steps.

The Twelve Steps of AA are not the only path to recovery support. Some people are uncomfortable in AA and related meetings. They may reject the notion of being "powerless" over their addiction. In fact, they may disagree with the entire concept of alcoholism as an addiction. Some are put off by the idea of appealing to a "higher power" and prefer to use only their own brains.

However, even people who did not attend "ninety meetings in ninety days," who don't continue to attend a weekly "home group" year after year, or who don't have a long-term relationship with an AA sponsor, rarely find fault with these principles. Even without a formal relationship with AA, most people with alternative, quality recovery programs actually use the same principles that are contained in the Twelve Steps. Here are some brief descriptions of some of these alternative approaches.

# Charlotte Kasl's 14-Step Program

Charlotte Kasl is a therapist who has worked extensively with women sex addicts and co-addicts. She consistently recommends to her clients that they attend twelve-step groups, but, in addition, she also recommends another model of recovery. In her book *Women, Sex, and Addiction: A Search for Love and Power* she describes a model that, over several years, will result in the gradual replacement of dysfunctional core beliefs with a set of true beliefs that lead to inner peace, healthy connections with other people, and a centered healthy sexuality. For years, women have gotten together in mutual-help groups to apply this model to their lives. Kasl's program is equally applicable to chemically dependent persons. Page 288 of her book gives the fourteen steps of her model:

1. Surrender: admit that you have problem.

2. Realize that you can't recover alone. Ask for help.

3. Be willing to do whatever it takes to recover.

4. Challenge your operational beliefs.

5. Identify your addicted and healthy sides.

6. Challenge the ways you reduce anxiety.

7. Use the addiction to grow.

8. Establish your definition of sexual sobriety.

9. Accept slips and recognize red flags.

10. Stay awake, stay aware.

11. Dive into your core beliefs and heal the inner child.

12. Learn new beliefs.

13. Acknowledge your spirituality.

14. Have a love affair with life.

You can see that the main elements of the Twelve Steps are included in this program—admitting powerlessness, asking for help, recognizing your unhealthy parts, making changes, monitoring your behavior, modifying your dysfunctional core beliefs, and doing this in the context of a spiritual life. In Step 5, Kasl makes the point that distinguishing between your addiction and the core of your being can help you to avoid unhealthy shame. If you experience an urge to use, tell yourself, "my addicted side wants to use," rather than, "I want to use." Tell yourself, "I am not my addiction" (Kasl, p. 296).

# Women for Sobriety (WFS)

In 1976 Jean Kirkpatrick founded an alternative program for women alcoholics. Kirkpatrick had relapsed after five years of sobriety during which she had attended AA. She proceeded to have a thirteen-year relapse, after which she recovered on her own. She wrote that this came about after realizing that she was a capable woman and that all her problems were the creation of her own mind. Kirkpatrick believed that women needed their own program of recovery, separate from AA. She created what she called a "New Life Program" that consisted of "Thirteen Statements of Positivity." At the time of her death in 2000 at the age of 77, there were more than 300 Women for Sobriety self-help groups in the United States, Canada, and several other countries. (See **www.womenforsobriety.org** for more information.) The thirteen affirmations of the program—originally written in 1976 and revised in 1987 and 1993—are listed below:

1. I have a life-threatening problem that once had me.
   *I now take charge of my life. I accept the responsibility.*
2. Negative thoughts destroy only myself.
   *My first conscious act must be to remove negativity from my life.*

3. Happiness is a habit I will develop.
   *Happiness is created, not waited for.*
4. Problems bother me only to the degree I permit them to.
   *I now better understand my problems and do not permit problems to overwhelm me.*
5. I am what I think.
   *I am a capable, competent, caring, compassionate woman.*
6. Life can be ordinary or it can be great.
   *Greatness is mine by a conscious effort.*
7. Love can change the course of my world.
   *Caring becomes all important.*
8. The fundamental object of life is emotional and spiritual growth.
   *Daily I put my life into a proper order, knowing which are the priorities.*
9. The past is gone forever.
   *No longer will I be victimized by the past, I am a new person.*
10. All love given returns.
    *I will learn to know that others love me.*
11. Enthusiasm is my daily exercise.
    *I treasure all moments of my new life.*
12. I am a competent woman and have much to give life.
    *This is what I am and I shall know it always.*
13. I am responsible for myself and for my actions.
    *I am in charge of my mind, my thoughts, and my life.*
    (c) 1976, 1987, 1993

To make the Program effective for you, arise each morning fifteen minutes earlier than usual and go over the Thirteen Affirmations. Then begin to think about each one by itself. Take one statement and use it consciously all day. At the end of the day review the use of it and what effects it had that day for you and your actions.

Again, you can see the similarities between the affirmations and the Twelve Steps. The differences are the increased stress on a woman's competence and her ability to make positive changes on her own, and a smaller emphasis on a higher power.

# Rational Recovery (RR)

An even greater emphasis on self-reliance and avoidance of appeal to a higher power is present in the nonreligious, abstinence-based program of Rational Recovery, founded in 1986 by Jack and Lois Trimpey as a for-profit organization. Jack Trimpey considered his program as an antidote to all the deficiencies he perceived in AA, and much of his speaking and writing was anti-AA. As explained in his book *Rational Recovery from Alcoholism: The Small Book* (usually called just The Small Book, in obvious contrast to the Big Book of AA), the founder of RR is actually Albert Ellis, whose Rational Emotive Therapy (RET) forms the foundation of the RR program. The RR program is "fast and simple; there are no 'higher powers,' no moral inventories, and no substitute dependencies or endless meetings to attend." (Trimpey, 1989, second edition, back cover). Instead, when you are tempted to drink, you need to remind yourself of the BEAST, which represents your addiction and is also a memory device for recovery. The acronym stands for:

> **B**oozing opportunity
>
> **E**nemy recognition
>
> **A**ccuse the beast of malice
>
> **S**elf-control and self-worth reminders
>
> **T**reasure your sobriety

Meetings are led by a professional or other person trained in the RR philosophy, the emphasis is on coping with urges, and members are expected to use their cognitive abilities to combat their desire to drink and to understand their slips. RR membership appears to have decreased in recent years, and it has been supplanted by SMART Recovery.

# Self Management and Recovery Training (SMART)

In 1994, a nonprofit group formerly affiliated with RR broke away from the Trimpey organization because members disagreed about the program of recovery to be offered in the self-help groups, and they changed its name to SMART. Like RR, SMART is a nonreligious, non-12-Step movement that is based on Albert Ellis' Rational Emotive Therapy (RET). SMART has a broader program than RR, one that includes attention to four points: motivation, coping with urges, problem solving, and lifestyle balance. (For more information, see **www.smartrecovery.org.**) Compared with the approximately 90,000 weekly AA meetings worldwide, SMART is still very small, having only about 250 meetings per week, nearly all in the United States.

Those of you who have had any addiction counseling following a relapse, or who are in relapse prevention, may be aware that standard relapse-prevention techniques in fact do employ techniques based on cognitive-behavioral therapy, which is the parent of RET. Cognitive therapy, according to Aaron Beck and his colleagues, "is a system of psychotherapy that attempts to reduce excessive emotional reactions and self-defeating behavior by modifying the faulty or erroneous thinking and maladaptive beliefs that underlie these reactions" (Beck et al., 1993, p.27). Behavioral therapy adds another piece—it focuses on changing self-defeating behaviors. The well-known relapse-prevention program of Terry Gorsky is a cognitive-behavioral one. Self-help programs like RR and SMART can be effective in relapse prevention, but they are less effective for newcomers to recovery, whose "best thinking" has often gotten them into trouble.

# Moderation Management (MM)

Moderation Management (MM) is a nonabstinence approach founded by Audrey Kishline in 1993. Its goal is to help problem drinkers reduce their drinking and make other positive life-style changes. Its audience is people who have experienced "mild to moderate levels of alcohol-related problems." MM promotes early recognition of risky drinking behavior, when moderation is an achievable recovery goal. MM is specifically *not* aimed at alcoholics. The basic text of the program is *Moderate Drinking: The New Option for Problem Drinkers*, written by Kishline in 1994. Unfortunately, Kishline eventually found that her own program was unable to help her control her own drinking, and in January 2000 she announced she was returning to AA, along with two other self-help alcohol recovery programs, and that she now realized that "moderation management is nothing but alcoholics covering up their problem." Two months later, in March 2000, while driving intoxicated on the wrong side of the road, she killed a twelve-year-old girl and the girl's father, and in July, Kishline was sent to prison for four and a half years. Meanwhile, the MM program continues to have meetings. (Source: **http://alcoholism.about.com/library/ weekly/aa000821a.htm**).

This sad story illustrates the basic problem with non–abstinence-based programs: A fundamental feature of addictive disorders is denial; addicts typically deny having lost control of their drinking or drugging, claiming, "I can always stop if I want to." This means that, although programs such as Moderation Management may indeed help someone who is drinking excessively but is not yet addicted, it is also likely to attract many addicts who are looking for the "easier, softer way." It is dangerous to trust your own judgment in terms of joining a "moderation" program, so this is not recommended.

Now that you have created a recovery support community for yourself, it is time to prepare a relapse-prevention plan. Chapter Ten explains how to do this.

## References

Alcoholics Anonymous World Services. *The AA Member-Medications & Other Drugs*. New York: Author, 1984.

Beck, Aaron T., Wright, Fred D., Newman, Cory F., and Liese, Bruce S. *Cognitive Therapy of Substance Abuse*. New York: Guilford Press, 1993.

Kasl, Charlotte. *Women, Sex, and Addiction: A Search for Love and Power*. New York: Ticknor & Fields, 1989.

Hamilton B. *Twelve Step Sponsorship: How it Works*. Center City, Minn.: Hazelden, 1996.

Kishline, Audrey. *Moderate Drinking: The New Option for Problem Drinkers*, 1994.

Trimpey, Jack. *Rational Recovery from Alcoholism: The Small Book*. Lotus, Calif.: Lotus Press, 1987.

# CHAPTER TEN: Relapse Prevention Planning

**prevent** v. *to act in anticipation of an event; to stop or keep from doing something*

**relapse** v. *to slip or fall back into a former condition after seeing improvement*

# How Relapse Happens

Relapse, like addiction, is a brain phenomenon. The frontal cortex (right behind your eyes) is the part of the brain that manages emotions, weighing reactions before acting. This part of the brain dampens the signals that urge us to instant action—fight or flight—when an emergency happens. The frontal cortex is like a parent who interrupts an impulsive child who is grabbing a cookie off a plate by asking her to wait until she's asked and received permission.

In earlier chapters we said that to stay sober you must be able to manage your emotional distress. Emotional distress is what triggers falling back on old ways of thinking and behaving. Once you become addicted, an emotional trigger and your old way of thinking makes you susceptible to what Daniel Goleman, author of *Emotional Intelligence* (1994), calls *an amygdala hijacking.* The distress is interpreted by the amygdala (a limbic center) as an emergency; it then switches off the signal that tells the cortex to stop and think before taking action. Emotional distress causes the brain to bypass that important emotional manager. That is why, when someone says "what were you possibly thinking?" when you went and bought crack and smoked all day instead of going to work, your reply is, "I don't remember" or "I wasn't thinking!" The emotional trigger or environment connected to an emotional event in the past opens up the pathway of least resistance, and that is where your addiction lives.

To avoid this vicious circle, you need to set up new ways, learn new skills, and keep yourself motivated and in balance. This is accomplished by completing and using a good a relapse-prevention plan. A valuable beginning is to see what challenges your sobriety right now.

# Sobriety Challenges

People who were raised in dysfunctional homes or who have been exposed to repetitive trauma or neglect learn toxic ways of responding to situations. These actions fall into four categories: withdraw, attack self, attack others, and avoid. Sometimes people rely on a combination of these actions. You can see them at work in the ways people argue with each other.

In arguments, generally something happens that triggers a vulnerable emotional state in people. They then shift into a toxic solution, usually reflecting what they have learned as children by watching their caregivers.

The first is blaming, arguing, and accusing. Another is to avoid any discussion and "stonewall" (i.e., withdrawing into silence—acting as if you could care less). In both cases, the vulnerable person might then revert to overreacting. The last method is to draw someone else into the discussion to lower one's anxiety and to create an alliance for an illusion of strength.

Initially these arguments can pump up your feelings of entitlement, resulting in defensiveness with those around you. This may leave you feeling angry or afraid, thinking you are flawed or a fool for being in the relationship, and behaving in ways that distance you or others from each other. Distancing behaviors usually result from being aggressive, saying something that is full of contempt or criticism, being passive-aggressive, or stonewalling. These anger actions are very damaging to relationships and can easily persuade you that you deserve to have that drink or to smoke that joint.

The underlying fear can result in passivity that leaves you feeling helpless, hopeless, and depressed. Once hopelessness sets in, feelings often get shut down, and isolation begins. This response is also an invitation to let go of your sobriety to try to alter your mood.

Besides reacting to relational problems, addicts challenge their sobriety in several other ways. Generally these manifest in extremes, either overdoing or not doing enough. For example, addicts often have a distorted sense of achievement: They will either complain all the time about not getting the break they deserve, or they overdo so much that they don't take care of themselves and create chaos in their lives. Often the addict either totally hides a secret life or is only minimally accountable, such as telling only what he or she believes someone else already knows. This may compromise self-esteem and lead to guilt and shame. Or else it can interfere with remorse so that the addict becomes self-absorbed by obsessions.

It takes self-awareness, specific skills, and motivation to stay out of these challenges and to maintain recovery. To be self-aware, you have to know what you are feeling and you must be able to manage negative thinking— that is part of tolerating emotional distress. Of course, in relationships it is helpful to have good communication skills, which include being assertive (not aggressive) in your communication efforts, giving and receiving positive feedback, listening, and taking and receiving criticism. Such skills make it easier to resolve problems in relationships.

Obviously, relationship problems and the inability to tolerate emotional distress are major triggers for sabotaging your sobriety. The following exercise pinpoints environments and situations that are particularly dangerous for you.

## Exercise 1:   Identifying High-Risk Situations

To be able to maintain your recovery, you have to be aware of the people, places, things, and emotions that will be high risk for you. Take a few moments to list the people that you either must avoid or learn to relate to differently. This might be old using friends that you have to stop seeing. Perhaps it is your mother-in-law who frequently triggers your anger and frustration; avoiding her in early recovery might be one solution. Then do the same with places or situations that you need to avoid or have a way to escape should you become triggered. You may need to avoid or change the way you handle certain things. These might include drug paraphernalia that you have hidden or might be exposed to in everyday life, or a hypodermic needle at the doctor's office. If you are an IV drug user, you might need a plan for dealing with urges that arise from seeing a syringe or hearing the nurse thump its side to get the air bubbles out. Finally, list the emotions that trigger you the most so you can make a plan to deal with them in a healthy way.

## People

_____

_____

_____

_____

_____

_____

_____

_____

## Places

_____

_____

_____

_____

_____

_____

_____

_____

## Things

_____

_____

_____

_____

_____

_____

_____

_____

## Emotions

_____
_____
_____
_____
_____
_____
_____
_____
_____

Review these lists and create five scenarios that are on the top-ten list of high-risk situations for you. Write those out below. Identify the skill you will need to handle the situation and how you think you can prevent or avoid the situation in the first place. (Skills are emotional, behavioral, or social in nature. These might be managing anger and negative thinking, using refusal or boundary-setting techniques, practicing positive thinking and visualizing desired outcomes prior to the situation, implementing a self-soothing alternative activity, listening more and repeating what you heard your partner say, visualizing negative consequences if you relapse, asking for help, asking how you can help the situation right now, being accountable and honest, or choosing not to carry cash.)

## Situation # 1:

_____
_____
_____
_____
_____
_____
_____
_____

*Skills needed:*

_____

_____

*How I might prevent or avoid the situation in the first place:*

_____

_____

## Situation # 2:

_____

_____

_____

_____

_____

_____

_____

_____

_____

_____

_____

*Skills needed:*

_____

_____

*How I might prevent or avoid the situation in the first place:*

_____

_____

## Situation # 3:

_____

_____

_____

_____

_____

_____

_____

_____

_____

_____

_____

_____

*Skills needed:*

_____

_____

*How I might prevent or avoid the situation in the first place:*

_____

_____

## Situation # 4:

_____

_____

_____

_____

_____

_____

_____

_____

_____

_____

*Skills needed:*

_____

_____

*How I might prevent or avoid the situation in the first place:*

_____

_____

**Situation # 5:**

_____

_____

_____

_____

_____

_____

_____

_____

_____

*Skills needed:*

_____

_____

*How I might prevent or avoid the situation in the first place:*

_____

_____

It will be helpful for you to think of as many high-risk situations as you can and make plans for how to avoid or escape them. Later we will come back to this exercise and use these situations to create emergency escape plans in case you are unable to avoid one or two of them.

You may have identified many skills that you don't yet have, or perhaps you were at a loss about what skills you would need. We have selected a few of the most important skills to learn, and we have put them in the relapse-prevention tool kit in the next section. Learning all these tools and talking with other addicts in recovery are essential for maintaining your sobriety. You will be surprised how helpful it is to learn refusal skills for when someone wants you to engage in a behavior that you want to stop. That is why practicing steps to stay sober and having a support group like a twelve-step group and a sponsor makes such a difference in your ability to cope. You may also need to learn how to manage any urges to drink or use another drug. In the past, using helped solve problems; in the present, you need to learn more effective ways to solve problems. One of these is to increase your list of pleasant activities to replace old behaviors that were not helpful in your sobriety.

Finally, it is critical for you to learn to manage anger and other emotional states and plan for emergencies. With all that in mind, let's begin to build a relapse-prevention plan by completing some exercises.

# Relapse-Prevention Tool Kit

This section contains several interventions and strategies that addicts have said helped them maintain their recovery. This is by no means a comprehensive list. If you find you are facing a high-risk situation for which you have no intervention planned, *ask for help*. First and foremost, strive for self-care and for balance in your life. We suggest you do the PCI for *at least six weeks* (twelve weeks is better) to help you get a rhythm or balance to your life. Additionally, you (and your partner if he or she is interested in learning this tool and using it to grow in the relationship with you) will want to complete a Thoughts and Feelings Journal every day for *at least four weeks* (again, doing this for ninety days is like magic for helping you learn how thoughts are connected to your emotions and what thinking errors you are making). Thoughts and Feelings Journal instruction starts on page 187. The Thoughts and Feelings Journal is a valuable tool in your tool kit.

## Exercise 2:   Counter Statements for Excuses to Use

Do you remember back in Chapter One we talked about the excuses you use to use? Review that exercise now, and use the excuses you identified through that exercise to complete this one. Transpose the twenty excuses from that exercise here, except this time compose a counter statement that takes the power out of that excuse. Here's an example:

Excuse to use: "I work hard, I just got paid, one little drink with my buddies won't be such a big thing. My wife will never find out. I can handle one drink."

Counter statements: "Yes, I do work hard and I agreed to bring home all the money and use only what we've budgeted for entertainment. One drink is too many for me because I am an addict and I can't stop with just one. My wife will find out, and she won't trust me anymore, and perhaps it will be the last straw. I want my sobriety and my wife. I can tell my buddies no thanks. "

Short version: "One drink is a relapse. It hurts me and the people I love and care about."

As you can see, for some people, thinking through each component of the excuse is helpful. For others, it is powerful to have it short, sweet, and to the point. See which style works best for you.

1.  Excuse:

   _____

   _____

   Counter statement:

   _____

   _____

2.  Excuse:

   _____

   _____

   Counter statement:

   _____

   _____

3.  Excuse:

   _____

   _____

   Counter statement:

   _____

   _____

4.  Excuse:

   _____

   _____

   Counter statement:

   _____

   _____

5.  Excuse:

   _____

   _____

   Counter statement:

   _____

   _____

6. Excuse:

_____

_____

Counter statement:

_____

7. Excuse:

_____

_____

Counter statement:

_____

_____

8. Excuse:

_____

_____

Counter statement:

_____

_____

9. Excuse:

_____

_____

Counter statement:

_____

_____

10. Excuse:

_____

_____

Counter statement:

_____

_____

11. Excuse:

_____

_____

Counter statement:

_____

_____

12. Excuse:

_____

_____

Counter statement:

_____

_____

13. Excuse:

_____

_____

Counter statement:

_____

_____

14. Excuse:

_____

_____

Counter statement:

_____

_____

15. Excuse:

_____

_____

Counter statement:

_____

_____

16. Excuse:

_____

_____

Counter statement:

_____

_____

17. Excuse:

_____

_____

Counter statement:

_____

_____

18. Excuse:

_____

_____

Counter statement:

_____

_____

19. Excuse:

_____

_____

Counter statement:

_____

_____

20. Excuse:

_____

_____

Counter statement:

_____

_____

## Exercise 3: Escape Plans

In Exercise 1, you identified high-risk situations to avoid. This exercise asks you to identify situations that might happen, which, despite your best efforts to avoid them, trigger you and put your sobriety at risk. For example, you go into your new boss's office at the end of the day. She tells you that one of her favorite activities is to review the day with her top management over a glass of wine. She has already poured you each a drink. What might be a couple of ways to escape this situation?

_____

_____

_____

What extreme measures would you be willing to use if your first attempts to escape did not work?

_____

_____

_____

List ten situations you might get into where you need an escape plan. These are not the same as the situations you want to avoid. Rather, they are situations you did not anticipate and have no control over. For each situation, list one or two ways to escape. Then list an extreme measure you'd be willing to take if the first two plans did not work.

1. Situation:

   _____

   _____

   _____

   Escape plan:

   _____

   _____

   _____

   Extreme measure:

   _____

   _____

   _____

2. Situation:

   _____

   _____

   _____

   Escape plan:

   _____

   _____

   _____

   Extreme measure:

   _____

   _____

   _____

3. Situation:

   _____

   _____

   _____

   Escape plan:

   _____

   _____

   _____

   Extreme measure:

   _____

   _____

   _____

4. Situation:

   _____

   _____

   _____

   Escape plan:

   _____

   _____

   _____

   Extreme measure:

   _____

   _____

   _____

5. Situation:

   _____

   _____

   _____

Escape plan:

_____

_____

_____

Extreme measure:

_____

_____

_____

6. Situation:

_____

_____

_____

Escape plan:

_____

_____

_____

Extreme measure:

_____

_____

_____

7. Situation:

_____

_____

_____

Escape plan:

_____

_____

_____

Extreme measure:

_____

_____

_____

8. Situation:

_____

_____

_____

Escape plan:

_____

_____

_____

Extreme measure:

_____

_____

_____

9. Situation:

_____

_____

_____

Escape plan:

_____

_____

_____

Extreme measure:

_____

_____

_____

10. Situation:

_____

_____

_____

Escape plan:

_____

_____

_____

Extreme measure:

_____

_____

_____

# Exercise 4:   Urge Reduction

When an addict gets triggered, it is common to experience an urge or a craving to use. The high-risk situations you identified previously all have the potential to trigger an urge response. It is important to know how to reduce the urge or craving to use. Obviously, an important strategy is to avoid or escape such situations. This exercise is adapted from the work of Peter Monti, a professor at Brown University. It is designed to help you identify things to say, think, or do that will help you "wait it out" when an urge hits you after you are triggered. Yes, "wait it out" is a part of what helps. If you can do something else that is healthy for fifteen minutes, your brain chemistry will change enough that the urge will usually subside—at least enough to call a sober friend or accountability partner.

Here are nine strategies that people use to get through urges or cravings.

1. Delay (fifteen minutes is usually long enough).
2. Thinking of negative consequences of using.
3. Thinking of positive consequences of sobriety.
4. Alternative behaviors.

5.  Reward for waiting out the urge.
6.  Meditation or formal relaxation methods.
7.  Escape or avoidance.
8.  Self-punishment.
9.  Willpower alone.

Research is clear that *self-punishment* and *willpower alone* do not work. In fact, self-punishment can grow into a form of altering mood and become addictive. Do *not* count on either to work.

The following are some examples that other addicts have used. Think about what you believe will work for you or that you have had some success with in the past. Under each heading, list several responses.

1.  Things I can say to myself to help me wait it out:

    "I can get through this. This urge will be less if I distract myself."

    "I am a strong man/woman in recovery. Recovery is my friend. I can wait this out."

    _____

    _____

    _____

    _____

    _____

    _____

    _____

    _____

    _____

2.  Negative consequences if I start to use again:

    My relationship with _____ will be in jeopardy.

    I will have to stay longer in treatment.

_____

_____

_____

_____

_____

_____

_____

_____

_____

_____

3.  Positive consequences of sobriety for me:
    Increased self-esteem.
    Relationship with _____ will have a better chance to improve.

    _____

    _____

    _____

    _____

    _____

    _____

    _____

    _____

    _____

4.  Healthy, pleasant alternative activities I can self-soothe or distract myself with:
    Take a walk and notice ten things I love in nature.
    Read a recovery book.

_____

_____

_____

_____

_____

_____

_____

_____

_____

_____

5.  Rewards for waiting it out:
    Increased self-esteem—evidence I am making progress.
    Read an escape novel.

_____

_____

_____

_____

_____

_____

_____

_____

_____

_____

_____

For which of the strategies was it most difficult to complete an extensive list? Which was the easiest? Most addicts find that thinking about healthy rewards or pleasant activities is very hard. On the other hand, thinking of the negative consequences for using is easy. What can you learn from your responses about which areas you will want to focus on in therapy or in discussing recovery with peers?

## Exercise 5:   Resolving Problems in Relationships

Relationship conflicts often trigger most addicts, but it is hard to avoid or escape your relationship if you want to keep it. It is not the relationship itself you want to avoid. As we have said many times before, the trigger is connected to unresolved problems that cause emotional distress.

Relationships are unique to the couple, so it is impossible to give you the solutions to all problems. Instead, this exercise is designed to help you think through the most common problems in your relationship and to take some practical steps that will help resolve the problems. Keep in mind that when problems come up, it is usually related to misunderstanding, incompatibilities, or some vulnerability related to unresolved childhood experiences. Some guidelines are helpful:

- No mind reading. Don't expect your partner to read your mind, and realize that you can't read your partner's mind. If you want to know something, ask.

- Don't let things that bother you build up. Try to give information about what is bothersome early on.

  - Calm yourself with deep breathing.

  - State how you feel when certain things happen (and if you know what childhood vulnerability it brings up, say so).

  - Speak about the specific behavior you want changed, rather than criticizing your partner as a person.

  - When asking for a change in behavior, ask for something that is clear and measurable. "I want you to love me more" is too vague. Instead, ask for some behavior that makes you feel loved.

  - Offer a compromise. Adults understand that we don't always get what we want in relationships. If you never get what you want after trying to resolve things, perhaps you need professional help.

- Express your positive feelings about the other person.
  - Compliment some behavior or effort you have noticed.

- Stick to the point. Talk about one issue at a time.

- Be an active listener.
  - Pay attention to the other person's feelings and vulnerabilities.
  - Ask questions.
  - Look at him or her.
  - Add comments or repeat back what your partner has said to show you have heard.

- Identify a "sacred space" for you as a couple in your home. Agree that the purpose of talk in this space is to help you as a couple and that it represents your commitment to try to heal and grow your relationship. Some people also hold hands or put both hands on some symbol that represents something sacred to both of them.

  Think about a current situation that is troublesome for you and your partner or another person. After you identify the situation, complete the following:

1. Describe the situation. (<u>Example:</u> I want sex more often than my partner wants sex.)

   _____

   _____

   _____

   _____

2. Describe what you usually do or fail to do in the situation that makes it worse. (<u>Example:</u> I hint to her that I am interested by nuzzling her neck or playfully pinching her behind. She frequently pulls away; sometimes she says mean things like "The only time you touch me is when you want sex." I then go and pout and don't pay any attention to her.)

_____

_____

_____

_____

3.  What would you like to try to do differently in this situation? (<u>Example</u>: I'd like to be able to talk to her about the differences in frequency and see what she'd like to do, so that when I want to just touch her because I care, I can.)

_____

_____

_____

4.  Now, choose the right time and place, and try out your new behavior or skill in the situation. Describe the results of the interaction and how your partner responded.

_____

_____

_____

Now repeat this process for the five most common problems you have with your spouse. A great resource for couples who want to do additional work is *Open Hearts*, by Deb and Mark Laaser. This workbook is available through Gentle Path Press.

## Exercise 6:   Twelve's List

On the next page, list twelve things you want to do every day that will help you maintain your recovery. Once the list is complete, make a few copies and put them in places (such as on a bathroom mirror or on the dashboard of your car) to remind you to do them. Some people put them on a card that they carry in their pocket. Over time, you will find that some things work better than others, so you will want to revisit this list occasionally with your therapist or sponsor and refine it. Some of the activities should reflect honoring your authentic self. Other self-care activities might include positive self-talk or daily affirmations, exercise, and healthy eating. Traditional recovery activities need to be included as well, including regular meeting attendance or calling your sponsor or someone else in your group. Relationship helpers might include being accountable and honest. Spiritual prayer or meditation is often listed. Staying aware of feelings by completing a Thoughts and Feelings Journal might be useful. You may want to write a long list on another piece of paper and then pick your favorite twelve.

1. _____

2. _____

3. _____

4. _____

5. _____

6. _____

7. _____

8. _____

9. _____

10. _____

11. _____

12. _____

## Exercise 7:   Emergency First-Aid-Kit

It also never hurts to have a little emergency first aid available. You can actually make yourself a *first-aid-kit* or box. Sometimes it is helpful to have several in specific places such as at home, in the car, or at the office. You can put things in the kit that remind you what your goals are for the future, who is important to you, evidence that you are a worthy person, and symbols that have meaning for you. You may even put some things on the outside of the kit or box to remind you what is inside. Some suggestions of things that others have found useful are:

- description of your authentic self

- a list of the values that guide you

- pictures of yourself as a kid and with those you loved

- pictures of those you love now

- favorite affirmations, meditations, prayers, and quotes

- phone numbers of support people

- tapes or CDs of special music

- symbols of recovery

- items that represent personal strength or accomplishments

- spiritual items

- letters or meaningful readings

- a fragrance you like (aroma oil)

One way to get beyond an urge is to look at the items in this box until your emotional distress changes. Take the time today to create your box. Below, indicate what you have included and how it will help you.

_____

_____

_____

_____

_____

_____

_____

## Exercise 8:   Relapse Contract

Now that you have some tools to use, it is time to make a commitment to your recovery. You can use the relapse contract as a way to talk to people who are important to you about what you will do if you do slip. You may want to make a copy of the contract for that other person and for yourself.

I (*your name*), _____, do agree that if I have a slip in my sobriety, I will do the following:

I will make every effort to limit what I have done and learn from the experience.

I will call you and let you know what my situation is.

I will also do the following [this should be what you and your sponsor, therapist, or accountability partner agree should be the first steps]:

_____

_____

_____

_____

_____

_____

_____

_____

_____

My sobriety date is: _____

Date of this agreement: _____

Signed, _____

This chapter has been devoted to creating your own personal relapse-prevention plan. More suggestions are listed at the end of the next chapter. Reread and readjust these answers every few months during the first two years of recovery. Use your plan to stop making excuses, avoid or escape high-risk situations, and continue to do what helps you be your authentic self.

While we think these skills are very important, we also know that slips and relapse are common in early recovery. Chapter Eleven tells you what to do if you have a slip or relapse.

## References

Hankes, L. Personal communication, 1999.

Laaser, Deb, and Mark Laaser. *Open Hearts.* Wickenburg, Ariz.: Gentle Path Press.

Monti, P., Rohsenow, D., Cooney, N., and Abrams, D. *Treating Alcohol Dependence: A Coping Skills Training Guide.* New York: Guilford Press, 2002.

# CHAPTER ELEVEN: Maintaining Long-Term Recovery

**maintain** v. *to keep up or continue*
**recovery** v. *to regain health, balance, and control*

# What to Do If You Have a Slip or a Relapse

First and foremost, if you have had a slip or relapse, don't give up. Learn everything you can from it. Go to more meetings, ask others for help, make amends, and be gentle with yourself. Guilt and shame are invitations to wallow in self-pity. Instead, keep moving and learning. A first place to start is with a slip or relapse autopsy.

## Relapse Autopsy

Just as a medical examiner looks closely at every part of a body during an autopsy to see what caused a person to die, we recommend that you regard your relapse in the same fashion. When considering the way your sobriety died, use some of the same tactics they use in TV crime programs that take a forensic look at crime scenes. They look at not just the body but also at all circumstances in order to determine what happened prior to the death. You will do the same when you autopsy your relapse.

Relapse does not begin with the drinking or drug use. It starts long before that in the ways you think, feel, and respond to events in your life.

It is also related to the people you are with, where you are, and how you manage your emotions. In order to prevent another relapse, it is critical for you to examine each thought and feeling you had and each action you took days and sometimes weeks before relapsing. If it is a slip, you still need to look at what led up to that behavior

Also examine your motivation. If you have lost the desire to maintain your recovery, revisit the problem and consequence list or take out your decision-making matrix again to see why you are looking for answers in all the wrong places.

People who are on the road to relapse usually do not reach out for help. If this is true of you, you probably think that no one can help you get through your pain or difficult situation. Instead, you tell yourself a lie—that no one is available to help. The truth is that you don't know unless you ask for help. If you ask, but the help that people offer isn't what you need, keep trying. Tell the person what you need—"I just need someone to listen," "I need you to come pick me up for a meeting," "I need you to suggest some things I can do to help myself here."

If you make a decision to use, relapse is virtually guaranteed. It is very hard to turn back once you tell yourself it is okay to use and once you commit to your addict self to do so.

All relapse is dangerous, but certain types of relapses are more problematic and represent a poor prognosis for long-term sobriety. One example is people who decide that as long as they're going to use, they might as well have an extraordinary "goodbye high." Unfortunately, this often results in an overdose or near-fatal outcome. Fantasizing about how good it is going to be, or how it will be better than any high you have ever had, is faulty thinking. It does not take into account the fact that, in the past, your tolerance built up gradually so you needed more of the drug in order to experience the same euphoria as when you began using. If you drink the same amount now, after a period of sobriety during which your tolerance has decreased, you are likely to have a blackout or experience alcohol poisoning, both of which can be dangerous. If you're using drugs, the same is true. More substance use equals greater toxicity and the greater likelihood of an unexpected overdose. If you are also engaging in high-risk behaviors to enhance the drug high, or vice-versa, you increase the odds that something bad will happen.

As much as you might want to blame others or circumstances for your relapse, ultimately you are responsible. The sooner you can take responsibility for making the choice to drink or use other drugs, the sooner you will be able to use the relapse as a learning experience. What you need to do now is focus on what triggered you and what you failed to do to increase your chances of staying sober.

Now for the autopsy and forensic exam. As odd as it may seem, it helps to start with the relapse or slip and work backwards in time. Reconstruct exactly what and how much you used and how you tried to cover it up or minimize your use, and identify who you lied to about using. (Don't forget to make amends for lying once you have completed the autopsy.) Continue going back in time, using your relapse-prevention plan (see Chapter Ten) as a guide to see where you failed to intervene with yourself and where you engaged in seemingly irrelevant decisions. For example, perhaps you decided to meet someone for lunch at what had been your favorite restaurant in the past, arrived a half hour early, and rationalized to yourself that they have such good food and that it is better to be early than late. If you don't have a relapse-prevention plan because you think you are sufficiently recovered not to need a plan to avoid or escape high-risk situations or thoughts, that is part of the problem. But this is not where the autopsy stops.

Continue to go back in time and record all the behaviors, thoughts, and feelings that led up to this relapse. Who were you seeing or talking to? Did something happen in the conversation that led to a feeling that then led to being emotionally triggered? Did you have a strong urge to use hours before you acted out? What kept you from telling someone or asking for help when you were triggered or were craving? When did you start to ignore or change the steps in your relapse-prevention plan? Did you ask anyone if it would be a good idea to make these changes? When did you start to lie to yourself? To others? When did you step over the line and decide it was okay to use?

Remember: During the first year or two of recovery, any changes in a relapse-prevention plan must be reviewed with your sponsor, accountability partner, group, and/or therapist.

Before relapsing, did you ignore signs that you were in trouble? Those signs are what help you know you need to go to more meetings, see your therapist, or talk with someone about the signs you are seeing. Remember that you need to monitor your disease, just as diabetics try to prevent relapse by checking their blood-sugar levels one or more times a day and adjusting their medication or diet as called for in their plan. If your addiction is feeling a bit out of control, do something about it.

Check out your environment. Did you adjust your behaviors to deal with triggers? If not, why? What excuses did you give yourself to rationalize not taking care? Did you go to old using places or see former using friends? Were you in touch with your feelings and did you work through them, or did you resume ignoring them, dissociating, and blaming others? Did you fool yourself by thinking that, if you had a good relapse-prevention plan and were truly working your program, you would not have another craving? Remember, your brain has been programmed to continue to crave your drug for quite some time after your last use. For some drugs, cravings last a long time. Craving is a normal part of the early recovery, so you must plan for it. (See urge reduction on page 232.) Have you suffered from the Lost Opportunity Syndrome? This syndrome is present when you have a chance to use with little chance of being caught—or the drug is just available—and, before you know it, you are telling yourself that you will really regret it if you don't use. This is a terrible thinking error and an extremely slippery area; it is a key reason for having an escape plan in place. (See page 227 for creating escape plans.) When you think you are done with your autopsy, put the work aside for a while, and then return to see if you might have missed something. If you had more than one relapse, do more than one autopsy. In all likelihood, you'll see a fairly consistent pattern with chronic recidivism, or tendency to relapse. If you find that you are having relapse after relapse, it may be that you are a likely candidate for long-term treatment. That means that you need to be in a safe environment in which it is hard to obtain your drug of choice. This break from your routine gives you the time to let your brain heal while you learn and practice new skills on a daily basis. Sometimes this means being in treatment for an extended period of time.

When you finish performing your relapse autopsy, reread it, beginning with the first trigger or feeling that started the ball rolling toward the decision to start using again. Look for the early warning stages that were present and that showed you were heading for relapse. The sooner you can identify early warning signs, the better your chances are for intervening before a significant relapse actually occurs.

Continue to learn and listen for early warning signs. Learn from every slip, and your relapses will be fewer and less severe.

# Increasing Your Levels of Care

When you relapse, it is helpful to increase your self-care. This can come in many forms, but here is a sample that was adapted from Dr. Lynn Hankes of the Washington State Physician's Health Program. The items here will give you an idea of how you might increase your level of care.

## Stages of Relapse and Recommended Action

**Stage 1. Early Relapse Symptoms:** Relapse thinking or behavior without chemical use, or specific acting out of behaviors that, as a part of your sobriety contract, you agreed to avoid.

**Action:** Increase the number of meetings you attend and check with your sponsor or accountability partner more often. Complete an inventory of behaviors and feelings that are signs of potential relapse. Review how to safeguard your environment, and catch and correct thinking errors. Sit with uncomfortable feelings, self-soothing in healthy ways until the emotional distress subsides. Review with others the positive consequences for remaining sober.

**Stage 2. Persistent Symptoms**: Persistent relapse thinking; relapse behavior without chemical use, such as lying. Life is out of balance.

**Action**: Increase the number of meetings you attend and check with your sponsor or accountability partner more often. Add an additional random drug screen and/or add a polygraph test. Demonstrate your ability to identify and correct thinking errors. Sit with uncomfortable feelings, self-soothing in healthy ways until the emotional distress subsides. Admit immediately when you've lied. Make amends where needed.

**Stage 3. Program Lapse Symptoms**: Persistent relapse thinking, good contact with program, brief chemical use, engaging in behavioral acting out such as work addiction or food addiction.

**Action:** Increase the number of meetings you attend and check with your sponsor or accountability partner more often. Add an additional random drug screen and/or add a polygraph test. Give your therapist permission to inquire of others about irritability, irresponsibility, inaccessibility, isolation, and other observations. Increase therapy. Restrict your behaviors and increase accountability to two sources that check with each other. Demonstrate your ability to identify and correct thinking errors. Sit with uncomfortable feelings, self-soothing in healthy ways until the emotional distress subsides. Admit immediately when you've lied. Make amends where needed. Review with two peers the negative consequences of relapse. Be accountable and make amends where needed.

**Stage 4. Partial Relapse Symptoms:** Relapse thinking and behavior, episodic or limited chemical use, some program contact but lying to peers about relapse dynamics.

**Action:** Increase the number of meetings you attend and check in with your sponsor or accountability partner more often. Add an additional random drug screen and/or add a polygraph test. Give your therapist permission to inquire of others about irritability, irresponsibility, inaccessibility, isolation, and other observations. Increase therapy or possibly enter residential treatment. Restrict your behaviors and increase accountability to two sources that check with each other. Demonstrate your ability to identify and correct thinking errors. Sit with uncomfortable feelings, self-soothing in healthy ways until the emotional distress subsides. Admit immediately when you've lied. Make amends where needed. Complete a relapse autopsy and change the relapse-prevention plan where needed. Review with two peers the negative consequences of relapse. Be accountable and make amends where needed.

**Stage 5. Relapse Symptoms:** Relapse behavior, more than episodic or limited chemical use, little or no program contact, isolation or overcompensating in other areas.

**Action:** Detox if needed. Have an assessment performed to determine if treatment or intensive outpatient program is necessary. In therapy or treatment, intensify accountability through behavioral contract and revisit decision-making matrix to determine motivation for continued sobriety. Review and modify one's relapse-prevention plan, and then determine the skills needed to implement the plan. Invite skills coaching in therapy. Complete and present a thorough relapse autopsy. If an outpatient, you should ask for an additional random drug screen and add a polygraph test. You should not return to work until you have successfully completed treatment or the therapist okays your return to work with specific guidelines for and restrictions needed at work. If an outpatient, increase accountability to two sources that check with each other. Demonstrate your ability to identify and correct thinking errors, implement an urge-reduction plan, and notify key people about relapse. Sit with uncomfortable feelings, self-soothing in healthy ways until the emotional distress subsides. Admit immediately when you've lied. Make amends where needed. Complete a relapse autopsy and change the relapse-prevention plan where needed. Review with two peers the negative consequences of relapse. Be accountable and make amends where needed.

**Stage 6. Relapse with Noncompliance Symptoms**: Full-blown relapse with extensive use, little or no program contact, does not respond to redirection.

**Action:** Detox if needed. You need to enter into long-term resident or inpatient treatment until treatment providers believe you are safe to return to home and work.

# Disclosure—an Ongoing Process

The subject of disclosing addiction secrets to your partner or family is very complex and is part of a lengthy process, one that begins for many addicts even before recovery. In fact, the first disclosure may be the event that gets an addict into recovery. For example, George's wife, Gloria, walked in on him one day as he was snorting cocaine in the bathroom. She had realized before this that George had recently changed in several ways and that he seemed unusually busy, but it was a shock to her to learn that he was addicted to cocaine. Over the next two days, they had many discussions about what was really going on. George admitted to her that he'd been using for a year, that he'd spent some of their savings to pay for the cocaine, and that the drug had revved up his sex drive so that he was spending a lot of time on the Internet downloading and viewing pornography. Gloria threatened to leave unless he got help for his addiction, and he did. Gloria stayed.

Other addicts go for addiction treatment, where they learn that rigorous honesty is an integral part of recovery, and only then do they disclose to their partner. In this situation, it is often possible to get a therapist to help with the disclosure.

The big issue with disclosure is that it usually involves admitting not only behaviors that are likely to upset one's partner, but also that there has been a lot of lying. Partners often report that learning about the lying was at least as bad as learning about the behaviors. Lying causes the partner to distrust the addict, which is why one of the key tasks when restoring the marriage or primary relationship is rebuilding trust.

How disclosure is initially done has a strong influence on how difficult the process of rebuilding trust will be. From a study on actual experiences of many recovering addicts and partners, we learned the following:

*When to disclose* is early on, before even more lies are told to cover up the behaviors. However, if you have a choice, don't just blurt out everything to an unprepared partner. Be sure that your partner has a support system to help her or him deal with the unwelcome information that you will be revealing.

*To whom to disclose* initially are the people who are most affected by your behavior, usually your spouse or significant other and other family members. If your work has been affected, you will need to disclose to your boss or supervisor. If you are in counseling and/or in a support group, you need to be honest with them.

*How much to reveal* initially is the broad outline of all your acting-out behaviors, but not the gory details. Some addicts attempt "damage control" by disclosing to the partner only what they believe she or he already knows. Others tell only what they think the partner will be able to handle, leaving out the worst behaviors. For example, a woman may admit to an affair but leave out that she is pregnant and doesn't know who the father is, or that this is only one of many affairs she's had. A man may admit to using cocaine but not that he was just arrested for selling drugs to an undercover policeman. The problem with this approach is that the partner is likely to find out the rest sooner or later, and she or he will then feel doubly deceived and even less inclined to trust the addict. Even though revealing all is frightening and risks bringing about the end of the relationship, there is no alternative if the relationship is to have any chance of surviving.

Some addicts do the opposite—in an attempt to relieve their guilt and have a fresh start, they tell their partner everything, every detail of their sexual acting out, every person they've bought drugs from or sold to or used with. Such "dumping" may fill the partner's head with intrusive images that are hard to forget, and it does not help the partner deal with the situation.

What is most helpful initially is to disclose enough so that the partner is not faced with major unpleasant surprises later on, but not enough to give graphic descriptions. It is important, however, to understand that even if the addict makes a sincere effort to reveal the extent of the acting out, additional disclosures may be necessary at a later time. Some reasons for not disclosing behaviors that occurred *before* recovery are:

- the addict may have forgotten some old behaviors,

- the addict may have been in an alcoholic blackout or drug-induced altered state and knows nothing about the behaviors,

- the addict may have said nothing about some behaviors or events because he did not think they were important,

- the addict may fear that the partner will physically harm him or her, or may believe that the partner is too ill or emotionally unstable to process the information.

# Disclosing a Relapse

One of the most difficult parts of a relapse, and one that keeps people in relapse dynamic, is disclosure about a relapse. Disclosure is a lengthy process because addiction is a relapsing disease. As we've discussed, many addicts have slips or relapses. Many partners (co-addicts) have their own distorted thinking, which includes believing that "if only I have all the information, I'll be able to prevent the problem, or I can control the situation." As they move ahead with their own recovery, they learn important lessons such as "I didn't cause the problem, I can't control it, and I can't solve it." Gradually they realize that knowing everything won't prevent a relapse, and it will only make them feel worse. They learn to set boundaries on what information they want to know and what they will leave to the addict to handle.

Couples need to discuss in advance the fact that slips or relapses might happen and how best to handle them. Some couples agree that the addict will disclose only behaviors that directly impact the relationship or that risk either partner's health. Examples include having sex with another person, or missing one's son's baseball game because the addict was hanging out with using friends. Other addictive thoughts and behaviors will be shared only with the therapist, sponsor, and twelve-step group. Sometimes partners also want to know where the addict is, psychologically. For example, if the addict is heading for a relapse, the couple agrees that the addict will tell his wife something like, "I'm really struggling now," and what he's doing about it, such as, "I'm talking it over with my sponsor and making some changes."

Partners who understand that relapse is a well-known risk of addiction are more likely to be empathetic if the addict does have a relapse and discloses it to them. Partners may still experience distress, anger, disappointment, and fear, but these emotions are likely to be less powerful if both people in the relationship have been communicating, if the addict has been honest in both small and large ways, and if the addict discloses sooner rather than later. Don't expect your partner or spouse to be instantly supportive and understanding. It may take her some time to feel her emotions and process them. If your partner is involved in her or his own twelve-step recovery program, she or he will have a support group with whom to express those feelings. Before you disclose, have in place your plan for learning from the relapse and preventing another, and sincerely commit to following through on it. When you do reveal the relapse, be sure to describe your plan and your commitment.

In summary, here are the steps for disclosing a relapse:

- Prepare in advance by discussing addiction and relapse with your partner.

- Disclose immediately if your partner's health is at risk as a result of the acting out.

- Don't wait a long time to disclose, but first discuss it with your therapist and sponsor.

- As part of the disclosure, describe what you have learned from the relapse and what you plan to do to prevent another one.

- Do not expect instant understanding and support from your partner. Give him or her some time to process the disclosure.

If you need additional information on disclosure to children, friends, and neighbors, and what to do about disclosing to others if you have legal problems, you can find more details in our book *Disclosing Secrets: When, To Whom and How Much to Reveal,* also available from Gentle Path Press.

# List of Skills to Learn for Long-Term Recovery

Although we have included several of these skills in Chapter 10, you might find it helpful to seek ways to learn these during your first two years of recovery. As research has repeatedly shown, these are the skills people find most helpful for maintaining recovery.

## *Skills for being in a relationship with oneself and others.*

Clarifying your values

Creating your authentic self

Developing good communication skills

    Nonverbal skills

    Conversation skills

    Listening skills

    Giving and receiving positive feedback or constructive criticism

    Learning to say "no thanks" or just plain "no"

    Asking for what you need; accepting that you may or may not get it

Self-soothing when emotionally distressed

Growing your relationship

Resolving relationship problems

Developing support networks

## *Skills for relapse prevention.*

Knowing your triggers, rituals, and high-risk environments to avoid

Identifying negative consequences of using

Identifying positive consequences for sobriety

Self-soothing when triggered by outside relationships

Reducing urges

Identifying thinking errors and seemingly irrelevant thinking

Managing negative thinking

Managing anger

Solving problems

Reducing stress

Practicing creative visualization

Planning for emergencies and creating escape plans

Increasing rewards for sobriety

Increasing self-enhancing and pleasant activities

Planning your short- and long-term goals

### *Tasks related to maintaining long-term recovery.*

Accepting that you have a problem

Understanding how your disease manifests itself in you

Establishing values

Creating and honoring your authentic self

Developing a spiritual life

Embracing the process of change and recovery

Learning to tolerate emotional distress

Limiting damage from your behavior

Establishing sobriety

Ensuring physical integrity

Participating in a community of mutual support

Reducing shame

Grieving losses

Understanding multiple and cross addiction and sobriety

Acknowledging the cycles of abuse and vulnerable brain chemistry

Bringing closure and resolution to addictive shame

Building supportive recovery relationships

Establishing balance, including healthy exercise and nutrition patterns

Resolving your original conflict wounds

Involving family members in therapy

Altering dysfunctional family relationships

Being an adult in relationships

Committing to recovery for each family member

Resolving issues with your children

Resolving issues with your extended family

Committing or recommitting to a primary relationship

Seeking validation from your inner self rather than from others

For more information related to these tasks, you might want to refer to *The Recovery Zone,* also available from Gentle Path Press and at **www.gentlepath.com.**

Congratulations! You are well on your way. We hope this workbook continues to be helpful for years to come. We wish you success on your road to recovery. Happy trails. Walk in sunshine.

## References

Hankes, Lynn, Levels of Relapse, Presentation at American Society of Addiction Medicine, 1999.

# APPENDIX A: Frequently Asked Questions on Drug Dependency, Treatment, and Recovery

## Q: What is drug-addiction treatment?

**A:** There are many classes of addictive drugs. Each addict's disease has specific features that require attention and characteristics that need to be taken into consideration. On the other hand, no addict's disease is theirs alone, and many who have found freedom through recovery have needed to overcome isolating themselves from others. Problems associated with drug addiction can vary significantly from addict to addict, and severity of addiction ranges widely.

Drug-addiction treatment can include behavioral therapy such as counseling or psychotherapy, medications, or their combination. Behavioral therapy offers strategies for coping with drug hunger and with triggers to drug seeking or drug use, relapse prevention, and problem-solving skills. When an addict's drug-related behavior places him or her at risk of infection with the human immunodeficiency virus and other infections, behavioral therapies can promote harm reduction. When an addict faces legal or financial problems, an attorney may be needed. When other mental disorders such as depression or if physical and sexual-abuse issues are present, mental-health services and medications may be needed to promote abstinence and rehabilitation. The best program for any given addict combines therapies and services needed while being flexible and sensitive to such issues as race, age, gender, sexual preference, pregnancy, employment, and current living conditions. Treatment may occur in a variety of settings such as out-patient programs. People with more severe problems often go to residential treatment for a period of time ranging from 30 days up to several months. Addicts who have to detox go to facilities like hospitals where medications can be administered and where professionals watch for medical stability. Because drug addiction is a chronic disorder characterized by relapses of differing frequency and severity, short-term one-time treatment often cannot be comprehensive enough to prevent the need for further interventions and renewed treatment.

## Q: Why can't addicts "just say no?" Why can't they quit on their own?

**A:** The abiding desire of nearly all addicts is to learn to be "responsible" or "social" substance users, able to stop using at will and on their own and without additional rehabilitation or major life changes. However, most of these attempts result in failure to achieve long-term abstinence. Research has shown that drug use over weeks or months, depending on the substance, results in significant changes in brain chemistry that persist long after the drug use has stopped. Some changes in brain function last for months or years after complete abstinence, whereas others appear to be permanent. Drug-induced changes in the brain of an addict directly alter perceptions of and desire to use the substance, alter the addict's ability to know when or to what extent he or she is "under the influence," and drive the compulsion to use more of the drug despite adverse consequences. Once such changes have occurred in the brain of a drug user, willpower is no longer sufficient to stop using, despite every logical reason to do so.

## Q: Why is drug-addiction treatment necessary?

**A:** Individuals in active addiction are in denial of the effects of their use upon themselves and others, and most often they are unable to make the changes in their lives that are necessary to maintain abstinence for extended periods of time, or to achieve meaningful recovery from substance addiction. The primary goals of treatment for the addict include:

- Acknowledging the problems associated with continued drug use.

- Learning skills for staying motivated for recovery and for maintaining recovery.

- Returning to effective functioning within the family, job or vocation, and the community.

- Reducing harm to self and others from substance use.

## Q: How effective is drug-addiction treatment?

**A:** Overall, statistics from outcome studies show that addiction treatment is at least as successful as the treatment of other chronic diseases, including diabetes, hypertension, and heart disease. A number of reliable studies have shown that drug treatment reduces substance use by 40 to 60 percent. Treatment outcome for any given addict will depend on the nature and severity of the presenting mental, physical, social, and legal problems; the appropriate matching of necessary treatment components; and the ability and extent of active, continuing engagement in the treatment process. The longer you have been an addict, the longer it takes to learn how to maintain long-term sobriety.

In terms of such measures as improvement in quality of life and productivity in the workplace and community, addiction treatment is extremely cost effective compared to alternative approaches such as law enforcement and legal and judicial services. According to conservative estimates, every dollar invested in addiction services saves between $4 and $7 in such costs, and it saves an equivalent amount in health-care related expenses and substance-related accidents. The annual cost of incarceration for drug-related crimes and social disorders is estimated to be approximately $18,400 per person.

## Q: What helps people stay in treatment?

**A:** Whether an addict is able to remain in treatment or not depends on factors associated with both the individual and the treatment program. A successful treatment outcome requires the addict to remain in treatment and to actively engage in the treatment process for sufficient time to make meaningful life changes. Individual factors related to engagement include motivation to change, degree of pain and suffering encountered prior to intervention, level of support from family and friends, and continuing pressure (often including the threat of further consequences) to remain in treatment from concerned parties including one's employer, criminal justice system, religious community, child protective services, or the family. Continuing care after completing primary treatment is especially important.

## Q: Why are 12 Step or self-help programs added to drug- addiction treatment?

**A:** Self-help groups can complement and extend the effects of treatment by professionals. They have been a basic part of both treatment and continued care for more than four decades. The most prominent and readily available groups are Alcoholics Anonymous (AA), Narcotics Anonymous, and Cocaine Anonymous, all based on the twelve-step model. AA has remained remarkably viable and practical for recovering addicts for more than sixty years. It takes some time and effort to find meetings that have particular appeal and meaning for any given addict. It is essential to find such meetings, establish a "home group" that is attended regularly, and secure a sponsor in the program who will work with the addict in early recovery on a regular basis. With such effort, a twelve-step fellowship becomes an ongoing and meaningful part of rehabilitation and long-term freedom from the tyranny of recurrent drug use following treatment.

One of the most common objections to participating in these groups is the belief that religion will be "pushed" on the recovering person. Twelve-step programs do encourage individuals to grow along spiritual lines but they do not proselytize or endorse any religious sect or denomination.

Alternative fellowships have been very helpful to some recovering addicts. Most treatment experts and recovering addicts consider involvement in some form of regular group activity that promotes recovery and supports abstinence from mood-altering substances to be essential for long term avoidance of relapse.

## Q: If an addict in recovery needs medication to reduce pain from an acute medical problem, can potentially addictive drugs be given safely?

**A:** Recovering addicts experience pain like everyone else. In the first hours or days of an acute medical illness, or during and following surgery, addicts will require equal if not higher doses of pain-relieving drugs, but they should be tapered off these agents as soon as possible. Home use of oral narcotics and other controlled substances that are prescribed for home use should be given in small quantities and their use monitored carefully. Addiction medicine specialists, certified by the American Society of Addiction Medicine or addiction psychiatrists who have earned a certificate of added qualifications (CAQ) in addiction, are available in most medical centers to provide guidance on the proper use of habit-forming drugs in recovering addicts during hospitalization or acute illness. Experience has shown that when such drugs are taken for relief of legitimate physical pain and quickly discontinued, the risk of initiating a relapse into addiction is low.

## Q: If an addict in recovery has a significant problem with chronic pain, can potentially addictive drugs ever be safely given?

**A.** Long-term treatment of *any* chronic pain patient with opioids (narcotics) is a last-ditch solution, after all other methods to either cure or alleviate the pain have failed. This includes surgery, physical therapy, exercises, injections into the painful area of local anesthetics and steroids by a specialist, and so forth. Anyone who is given more than small doses of opioids for more than a few weeks usually becomes *physically dependent* (meaning they will experience withdrawal symptoms if they stop suddenly), but chronic-pain patients who have no prior addiction history are unlikely to become *psychologically addicted*. On the other hand, people with addiction histories, especially those with a history of narcotic addiction, are at increased risk of addiction. If potentially addictive drugs are prescribed to them, it should be under strict monitoring, and the patients need to intensify their recovery activities. Untreated drug-dependent persons are not candidates for such drugs for pain management because they cannot use the drugs responsibly.

## Q: How common is drug dependency?

**A:** Alcohol dependence and related drug dependencies have become so common that most people are aware of one or more people from their family, social network, work environment, or community of faith, who have struggled with drug or alcohol addiction. Within the last two decades, many experts in the diagnosis and treatment of addictions have observed a definite increase in the number of mood-altering substances that a patient presenting for treatment has tried. They have also noted an increase in the number of those substances that have been used by the patient to fulfill the clinical criteria needed to make the diagnosis of dependency.

More than half of current U.S. residents aged 18- to 58 have used marijuana or some other illicit controlled substance at least once. The majority have also smoked tobacco or used it in some other form. An even higher percentage has consumed alcohol. Out of every three persons who have smoked tobacco, one has active nicotine dependence. Out of every seven persons who have consumed alcohol, one will develop alcohol dependence. And, out of every seven people who have used an illicit controlled substance at least once, one has become dependent on a controlled substance at some point in his or her life (Anthony et al., 1994).

## Q: What does the term *dual diagnosis* mean?

**A:** *Dual diagnosis* refers to the concurrent presence of both drug dependency and other mental disorders such as major depression, bipolar disease, or anxiety. Mental disorders increase the risk of either developing drug dependence or exacerbating a preexisting drug addiction. Treating the psychiatric disorder in most circumstances does not treat the substance dependency, and vice versa. Not treating the psychiatric disorder increases the risk that addicts will either avoid committing to the treatment process, drop out of treatment early, or relapse back into active addiction.

## Q: My family is concerned about my drinking *but* I only drink on the weekends and I never have difficulty functioning at work. How can I possibly be considered an alcoholic?

**A:** Even if you do not believe that your use of alcohol has created consequences, someone in your family does. Their concern is a problem for you until you are able to understand *why* they are concerned. Take the time to sit down with them and ask them why they have such concerns. Perhaps the information on which they are basing their concerns is incorrect. Perhaps they can see your use of alcohol creating difficulties that you have not been able to recognize on your own. You probably have much more to lose by avoiding the issue than by addressing it with your family.

The fact that you have not experienced difficulty functioning at work should be of limited comfort to you. This is a poor rationalization to make in order to prove to your family that your weekend drinking is not a problem. Virtually all major studies on the natural history of alcoholism show work performance is the last area in an alcoholic's life to be affected. Moreover, an addiction is not determined nor classified on how often you use, but rather on what happens when you do use. Even if you drink only once a month, but you black out and cannot function without the alcohol, you still can be considered an alcoholic. For an infrequent user, drug dependency can also be characterized by how thinking about drug abuse affects your life—for example, if you are spending a lot of time thinking about your supply of drugs. When your activities are centered around drug abuse, it changes your mood and behavior and can isolate you from others. If you continue to use after these consequences, even if it's only on weekends, you are experiencing addiction/drug abuse problems. It is important to listen to your friends and loved ones; they often see something within ourselves that we are either too afraid or too detached to even acknowledge.

## Q: My daughter has started smoking cigarettes. Even though I am not terribly concerned, my husband is afraid that nicotine can lead to other addictions and dangerous habits. Who is right here?

**A:** Your husband is correct. It is a misconception to believe that soft drugs, such as nicotine, are not a gateway to hard-core drugs. Nicotine or marijuana addiction may lead to another addiction. The truth of the matter is that nicotine and cannabis are addictions that need to be addressed and acted upon. Cigarette smokers are significantly more likely to use other drugs than are nonsmokers, and we know that nicotine addiction kills more people each year than all other drugs combined. Cigarette smoking can be a gateway for other drug usage because it sets up a rationalization and pattern of denial in the addict's thought process, so the addict is more likely to act similarly toward other drugs. In most societies, the sale of cannabis is not legal. People who engage in one illegal activity are more likely to engage in other illegal activities as well.

## Q: What is the difference between bingeing and controlled, episodic use? I smoke/drink several times a month, but it's never on a particular day or set schedule.

**A:** Chronic addiction problems develop over time, and everyone has a different maintenance level. Some people can be drinkers for fifteen years before they question if they have an addiction problem. The bottom line is that controlled use is a different type of addiction than bingeing. Planned or at least premeditated social substance use in a responsible manner where there are no harmful effects or consequences for yourself or others may be a reasonable life choice for a person, if done in moderation. When episodic use begins to cause harm or consequences, then it is time to recognize that you have stepped over the line from controlled episodic use to bingeing, even if there are only a few occasions that you can identify when your use was excessive. Unfortunately, even "controlled" use of some substances can lead to addiction and profound consequences to health and well being, especially when this use becomes a ritualized pattern that is maintained over months or years. Dr. Robert Dupont, author of *The Selfish Brain,* states that healthy social drinkers do not drink more than two drinks in a twenty-four hour period or four drinks in a week. He states that if you are drinking more than four drinks in a twenty-four hour period or more than ten drinks a week, you are at risk for serious alcohol-related problems. Those who drink five or more drinks in a twenty-four hours period or more than ten drinks a week are showing presumptive evidence of a serious drinking problem. (A drink is defined as twelve ounces of beer, five ounces of wine, or 1.5 ounces of distilled spirits.)

## Q: Is it right or wrong to ask someone to take a drug test?

**A:** Urine drug screens are laboratory tests that can be helpful in the diagnosis or treatment of substance addiction. It is neither right nor wrong to ask someone to submit to a test. When you consider asking someone to produce a sample for urine drug screening, it is important to review your reasons for making the request. If the test is required as part of pre-employment evaluation, or to assure public safety, as required by certain professions or the Department of Transportation, it should be presented as a necessary part of employment and public (or company) policy.

When you are concerned about possible drug use by someone in your family, someone you love, or a close friend, it is best to request a urine drug screen only under very clear circumstances. It may be appropriate to do so as part of an intervention, following an accident involving the family car or boat, or as part of an addiction-recovery program under the supervision and direction of a professional.

## Q: When my partner uses drugs and drinks alcohol, I do not feel safe because his behavior becomes violent. How do I handle it? What do I do?

**A:** Domestic violence, spouse abuse, and battering all refer to the victimization of a person with whom the abuser has had an intimate relationship. Domestic violence may take the form of physical, sexual, and psychological abuse, is generally repeated, and often escalates within relationships. The prevalence of domestic violence in North America is staggering and difficult to fully appreciate. Nearly one-quarter of women in the United States are abused by a current or former domestic partner within their lifetime. Battery is the single most significant cause of injury to women in the United States. However, only about one in twenty (5 percent) who enter the health-care system have the cause of their trauma correctly identified as spouse abuse. Batterers came from all socioeconomic groups, cultural backgrounds, and sexual orientations. Domestic violence is far more than a single episode of trauma. Approximately 47 percent of husbands who beat their wives do so three or more times a year. Rape is a significant or major form of abuse in more than half of violent marriages. Among battered women who are first identified in a medical setting, more than three out of four will go on to suffer repeated abuse. Government sources estimate that between 2 and 4 million domestic partners will be physically assaulted by their spouses or living partners this year, and that 2 to 4 thousand of them will die as a result of battering.

Domestic violence and family violence are associated with drug abuse and drug addiction. Men who have assaulted their female partners are more likely to have witnessed or experienced violence in childhood, to abuse alcohol, to be sexually assaultive toward their partners, and to be at risk for perpetration of violence against their children. Not only is domestic violence perpetrated by the alcoholic spouse on the sober spouse, it is also inflicted on the alcoholic spouse by the sober spouse. Not all batterers drink. The "drunken bum" theory of wife beating tends to relieve the batterer of responsibility and to imply that violence will cease with abstinence. Alcohol or drugs may be used to rationalize violent behavior. Perpetrators and family members may insist that drug abuse is the problem. Evidence indicates that, although substance abuse and violent behavior frequently coexist, the violent behavior will not end unless interventions address the violence as well as the addiction.

Remember that abused partners need to acknowledge not only the violence and pain they are experiencing but also the difficulty they may have in escaping from abuse. Many abused spouses have limited options. If a battered spouse chooses to continue in the relationship, the risk of further intimidation, if not continued episodes of violence, is great, even with counseling. Yet, if the battered spouse leaves the residence, what financial, legal, and support resources will be available for the family? If domestic violence is reported and even if a restraining order is obtained, will it prevent further threats? How will the family bills be paid if the batterer is forced to leave?

For many battered spouses and their families, there are no easy answers, but there is hope. Many perpetrators are seeking help for their anger and violent behavior. In time, we may establish shelters for the batterers as well as for the battered. Therapy can and does make a difference. Early identification of the cycle of violence may limit its spiral into serious physical and emotional trauma, and it may help prevent yet another generation from living through the pain of this fateful struggle that goes on behind closed doors.

## Q: My friend acted totally out of character and said some very embarrassing things at a party we went to. We were both drinking, but when I confronted her with what she said and did she had no recollection or memory of behaving that way.

**A:** One of the more common symptoms of addiction and abuse is the use of a substance to a point where you do not remember. This is also called a *blackout*. People have different tolerance levels, and blackouts can happen at any particular time. However, a blackout is of particular concern because it represents a period of amnesia—that is, many minutes or hours of time under the influence of a substance, which cannot be accounted for or remembered. In some respects, it represents a state of anesthesia while still walking and talking! The person who experiences a blackout typically does not recognize the danger and consequences of a blackout. A blackout clearly signifies progression in the severity of drug dependency. "Social" users, and even abusers of alcohol do not experience blackouts. A blackout is convincing evidence that a person has a serious drug dependency. It is very frustrating to try to convince someone of what they said or did during a blackout. The best way to approach someone who may deny the signs or behavior associated with a blackout is to confront them over words or actions that have been witnessed by more than one person. Another effective technique is to confront the person with a course of action that they cannot remember doing yet know they have done, such as driving home. It is also important not to blame or excuse the drug as the reason for a person's behavior. If, once you begin abusing a drug, you cannot determine whether or not the use will result in behavior problems or a blackout, these are clear indications you have progressed from drug use or abuse to drug dependency

**Q:** **While I was putting my son's laundry away, I found a marijuana cigarette hidden under his socks. I don't want him to think I am a nosy parent and I don't want my son to think that I was invading his privacy, but I don't know what to do.**

**A.** Finding any kind of evidence of illicit drug use by your child, even a marijuana cigarette, definitely represents a significant opportunity to intervene. It provides an opportunity to "raise the bottom" by creating consequences for use at this point rather than at a later point, such as when your child is discovered driving a car under the influence of marijuana. If you choose not to intervene, you are passively or indirectly consenting to his use of marijuana and supporting his drug use. *Parents have not only a right but an obligation to address and remove any hazards or dangers to the safety and well-being of their children.*

You have a responsibility as a parent to be aware of safe and unsafe things in your house. You wouldn't think twice about controlling any guns in the house, or a chemical agent like rat poison, so why should drugs be any different? The "invasion of privacy" argument from a child is a common response to this situation, but by no means is this an invasion of your son's privacy. *As the responsible adults in your child's life, it is your responsibility to confront any threats to your child's welfare.* It is your job to know what is happening in your child's life. If your child already knows that his behavior is against the rules, then you have to be consistent and support those rules. Finding any kind of evidence should set off a red light in your head. Illicit drug possession is considered evidence of illegal drug use until proven otherwise. Illicit drug possession may result in legal consequences that are far more serious than the assertion of parental rights and the pain of parental consequences.

When you must confront an adolescent about a discovery, try to pick a time when he or she is not with their friends. Choose a time when all parental figures can sit down with the individual and express their concern. At the beginning of the discussion, ask the adolescent to listen to what everyone has to say. Assure them that they will have the opportunity to respond after everyone else has spoken. Try to use language that shows concern and is not judgmental. Avoid anger and shouting, and do not make any threats you are not willing to undertake. If you do not feel confident in conducting the intervention, then seek some assistance from an addiction counselor who can prepare you for the confrontation. Finally, have all parental figures who are involved agree by consensus on acceptable outcomes and consequences of the meeting. Drug abuse is very serious and can escalate very quickly.

# APPENDIX B: Resources

## Twelve-Step Programs—Contact Information

### Adult Children of Alcoholics

P.O. Box 3216

Torrance, CA 90510

Tel. (310) 534-1815

Web site: **www.adultchildren.org**

### Alateen

Alateen, Al-anon Family Group Headquarters

P.O. Box 862, Midtown Station

New York, NY 10018-0862

Web site: **www.al-anon.alateen.org**

**Alcoholics Anonymous World Services**

P.O. Box 459, Grand Central Station

New York, NY 10163

Tel. (212) 870-3400

Email: **WSO@alcoholics-anonymous.org**

Web site: **www.alcoholics-anonymous.org**

**Al-Anon World Services Office**

1600 Corporate Landing Parkway

Virginia Beach, VA 23454-5617

Tel: (888) 4AL-ANON

Email: **WSO@al-anon.org**

Web site: **www.al-anon.alateen.org**

**Cocaine Anonymous World Services**

P.O. Box 2000

Los Angeles, CA 90049-8000

Tel. (310) 559-5833 or (800) 347-8998 (meeting information)

Email: **cawso@ca.org**

Web site: **www.ca.org**

**Co-Dependents Anonymous**

P.O. Box 33577

Phoenix, AZ 85067-3577

Tel. (602) 277-7991

Web site: **www.codependents.org**

**Dual Disorders Anonymous**

P.O. Box 4045

Des Plains, IL 60016

Tel. (708) 462-3380

**Emotions Anonymous**

P.O. Box 4245

St. Paul, MN 55104

Tel. (651) 647-9712

Web site: **www.emotionsanonymous.org**

**Narcotics Anonymous World Service, Inc.**

P. O. Box 9999

Van Nuys, CA 91409

Tel. (818) 773-9999

Email: **wbmail@na.org**

Web site: **www.na.org**

**National Council on Sexual Addiction and Compulsivity**

P.O. Box 725544

Atlanta, GA 31139

Tel. (770) 541-9912

Web site: **www.ncsac.org**

**Overeaters Anonymous**

P.O. Box 92870

Los Angeles, CA 90009

Tel. (310) 618-8835

Web site: **www.oa.org**

**Women for Sobriety**

P. O. Box 618

Quakertown, PA 18951

Tel. (215) 536-8026

Web site: **www.womenforsobriety.org**

## Twelve-Step Reading

Al-Anon Family Group Headquarters. *Al-Anon's Twelve Steps & Twelve Traditions.* New York: Author, 1981.

Alcoholics Anonymous World Services, Inc. *Twelve Steps and Twelve Traditions.* New York: Author, 1952.

Alcoholics Anonymous World Services, Inc. *Alcoholics Anonymous, 3d ed.* New York: Author, 1976.

Alcoholics Anonymous World Services, Inc. *Living Sober.* New York: Author, 1975.

Alcoholics Anonymous World Services, Inc. *Alcohólicos Anonimos.* New York: Author, 1990. [The Big Book in Spanish]

Hamilton B. *Twelve Step Sponsorship: How it Works.* Center City, MN: Hazelden Information and Services, 1996.

Philip Z. *A Skeptic's Guide to the 12 Steps.* Center City, MN: Hazelden Information and Services, 1990.

World Service Office, Inc. *Narcotics Anonymous, Fifth Edition.* Van Nuys, CA: Author, 1988.

## Other Helpful Reading

Beattie, M. *Codependent No More.* Center City, MN: Hazelden, 1987.

Beattie, M. *Beyond Codependency.* Center City, MN: Hazelden, 1989.

Fossum, M.A., and Mason, M.J. *Facing Shame.* New York: W.W. Norton & Company, 1986.

Goleman, D. *Emotional Intelligence*. New York: Bantam Books, 1994.

Gorski, T.T. *Passages through Recovery: An Action Plan for Preventing Relapse*. Center City, MN: Hazelden, 1989.

Gorski, T.T., and Miller, M. *Staying Sober: A Guide for Relapse Prevention*. Independence, MO: Independence Press, 1986.

Larsen, E. *Stage II Recovery: Life Beyond Addiction*. Minneapolis, MN: Winston Press, 1985.

Miller, M., and Gorski, T *Learning to Live Again*. Independence, MO: Independence Press, 1980.

Peck, M.S. *The Road Less Traveled*. New York: Simon & Schuster, 1978.

Rustin, Terry. *Quit & Stay Quit: A Personal Program to Stop Smoking*. Center City, MN: Hazelden, 1991.

Trimpey, Jack. *Rational Recovery from Alcoholism: The Small Book*. Lotus, CA: Lotus Press, 1987.

# Twelve Steps of Alcohol Anonymous

Generally, most people complete the Twelve Steps with a sponsor. Using the answers to the questions in this book, you will find it easier to complete any assignments your sponsor may give you to complete the Twelve Steps. The Steps are listed below:

1. We admitted we are powerless over alcohol—that our lives had become unmanageable.
2. Came to believe that a Power greater than ourselves could restore us to sanity.
3. Made a decision to turn our will and our lives over to the care of God as we understood Him.
4. Made a searching and fearless moral inventory of ourselves.
5. Admitted to God, to ourselves, and another human being the exact nature of our wrongs.
6. Were entirely ready to have God remove all these defects of character.
7. Humbly asked Him to remove our shortcomings.
8. Made a list of all persons we had harmed, and became willing to make amends to them all.
9. Made direct amends to such people wherever possible, except when to do so would injure them or others.

10. Continued to take personal inventory and when we were wrong promptly admitted it.

11. Sought through prayer and meditation to improve our conscious contact with God as we understand Him, praying only for knowledge of His will for us and the power to carry that out.

12. Having had a spiritual awakening as the result of these steps, we tried to carry this message to others, and to practice these principles in all our affairs.

# Thoughts–Feelings Journal

Date_____

## Event or situation

_____

_____

_____

## What happened?

_____

_____

_____

## Who was there?

_____

_____

_____

## When and where?

_____

_____

_____

## Thoughts

What thoughts were going through your head just before the event, during the event, and immediately after the event? Circle the thoughts that may be related to your core beliefs about yourself.

_____

_____

_____

_____

_____

_____

_____

_____

_____

### Emotions

What emotions did you feel? Underline the strongest two feelings. Circle feelings that are triggers for you to want to act out.

_____

_____

_____

### Body sensations

Often the body gives us a signal that something is going on before we are really aware that we may be in a bad place. Listen to your body. Describe any body sensations you felt during the process.

_____

_____

_____

What does your body do when you get angry or sad?

_____

_____

_____

How does it tell you that you are having a strong feeling or reaction?

_____

_____

_____

### What I did well

_____

_____

_____

When we've gotten into a highly emotional situation that we've mismanaged, we think we made a mess of everything. This section is to remind you
that you did do something right (usually). Think about what part of the
situation you handled well or did not make worse. Note those items here.

_____

_____

_____

## How I made things worse

In this section, list the ways you made the situation worse.

_____

_____

_____

## Thinking errors

Look at your thoughts from section 2 (Thoughts) of this journal entry. Are
any of those thoughts thinking errors? Actively search for information or
evidence that contradicts the thoughts or that supports the thoughts.

_____

_____

_____

_____

_____

_____

_____

_____

_____

_____